The Prevention of
FOOD POISONING
2nd Edition

Spores - Bacillus & Clostridium

Also published by Stanley Thornes

P A Alcock   *Food Hygiene: A Study Guide*

Janet Hughes and Brian Ireland   *Costing and Calculations for Catering*

Julia Reay   *A Guide to Catering Organization*

Chris Ryan   *An Introduction to Hotel and Catering Economics*

Iris Jones and Cynthia Phillips   *Commercial Housekeeping and Maintenance*

Lilian M Gawthorpe   *Food and Nutrition; Family Meals*

Doug Kincaid and Peter S Coles   *Science in a Topic: Food*

The Prevention of FOOD POISONING

2nd Edition

Jill Trickett MSc

Senior Lecturer in Food Hygiene
Salford College of Technology

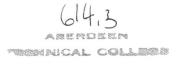
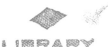
Stanley Thornes (Publishers) Ltd

2101-3

First published in 1978 by:
Stanley Thornes (Publishers) Ltd
Old Station Drive
Leckhampton
Cheltenham GL53 0DN

Reprinted 1980, 1982, 1984, 1985
Second edition 1986
Reprinted 1987
Reprinted 1989
Reprinted 1990
Reprinted 1991

Tricket, Jill
The prevention of food poisoning.—2nd ed.
1. Food poisoning
I. Title
615.9′54   RC143

ISBN 0-85950-613-4

Text set in 11/13 pt Italia by Tech-Set, Gateshead, Tyne and Wear.
Printed and bound in Great Britain at The Bath Press, Avon.

Contents

Preface to the first edition

My aim in writing this book is quite simply to provide an introduction to the subject of food poisoning. The fact that the number of outbreaks of food poisoning is increasing each year despite apparently higher living standards and high standards of personal hygiene suggests that many staff employed in the catering industry, and many housewives, have no knowledge of the causes and prevention of food poisoning.

The book seeks to offer an interesting and logical approach to the basic principles of bacterial growth with special emphasis on pathogenic bacteria, their sources, means of access to the kitchen, ways of controlling their growth in foods and hence the prevention of food poisoning. No previous knowledge of the subject is required but for anyone already acquainted with the basic ideas, the provision of sub-headings should make it possible to refer to any particular subject area.

The need for such a book was brought home to me while preparing a course of lectures on food hygiene for students taking the Royal Institute of Public Health and Hygiene's certificate examination in Food Hygiene and the Handling of Food. It seemed to me that there was not a suitable book for students at this level, the majority of textbooks being too advanced for the requirements of the course. In addition I hope it will be useful for students taking A level GCE Home Economics papers, and for those taking City & Guilds of London Institute Catering Courses. Above all, I hope that the general reader will find much of interest.

J. Trickett

Preface to the second edition

Since the appearance of the first edition there have been several new developments in the field of food hygiene which deserve a mention in a book of this nature. In particular, the increasing use of specialised equipment for catering (such as microwave ovens, cook-chill and cook-freeze systems) makes it important to include a consideration of the hygiene aspects of its use. Details of several other causes of food poisoning and food-borne diseases have been added. Those which occur relatively infrequently have been included in the appendices.

Several new courses and examinations are now being offered by various bodies concerned with hygiene and the food industry, and I have expanded the contents of the book to cover syllabuses while maintaining a readable text for those who are not taking examinations but merely wish to understand the principles of the prevention of food poisoning.

J. Trickett   June 1986

Acknowledgements

My sincere thanks go to: Mr R. R. Charnock of The College, Swindon who first suggested that I should write this book; and to him and Mrs B. D. Martin who read the manuscript making a number of suggestions.

Mr D. Harley and Mr B. Mallett of the Public Health Laboratory, Southampton General Hospital for preparing slides and to the Department of Teaching Media, Southampton General Hospital who prepared the photographs.

Dr A. C. Buck, consultant pathologist, Princess Margaret Hospital, Swindon for providing further slides.

Mr R. Moore, formerly Superintendent Food Safety and Hygiene Officer, Sheffield, and Mr M. S. Wildsmith, senior Public Health Inspector, Thamesdown for their help with technical data.

My parents for checking through the manuscript, and Mrs W. E. Greenway for typing it.

I am grateful for the help received from Rentokil Ltd (photographs on pages 96, 97, 99, 100), Clenaglass Electric Ltd (reference for illustration on page 84), Haigh Engineering Ltd, Pifco Ltd, Sissons of Sheffield (reference for illustration on page 92), London School of Hygiene and Tropical Medicine and Science Photo Library (photograph on page 20), Dr Tony Brain and Science Photo Library (photograph on page 25), CNRI and Science Photo Library (photograph on page 29), and Miss M. A. Munford of Marks and Spencer PLC whilst putting together the second edition. Thanks are due to The Community Disease Surveillance Centre for permission to use their figures and to The Health Education Council for permission to reproduce their posters; also to Dr Helen Whitwell for her help with photographs and to my husband Stuart for his help in many ways.

Thanks are due for permission to reproduce questions from past examination papers to the Royal Society of Health, the Associated Examining Board and the University of London Examining Board.

Cover illustrations: Anthony Blake Photo Library, London School of Hygiene and Tropical Medicine and Science Photo Library, Dr Tony Brain and Science Photo Library, and Mr T. Moran.

Chapter 1

Introduction to Bacteria

Bacteria are so small that they can be seen only through a microscope. A bacterium has a very simple structure consisting of one cell only whereas the human body (or that of any animal or insect) is made up of countless numbers of different cells.

Approximately one million bacteria clumped together would cover a pin-head. There are many different types of bacteria and they vary in shape and size but the ones found in food are usually spherical (*cocci*), rod-shaped (*bacilli*) or comma-shaped (*vibrios*).

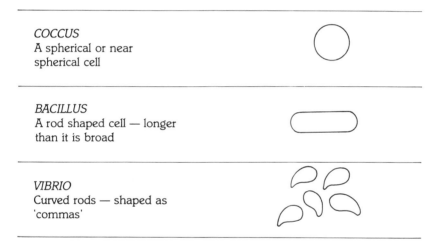

COCCUS A spherical or near spherical cell	
BACILLUS A rod shaped cell — longer than it is broad	
VIBRIO Curved rods — shaped as 'commas'	

Bacteria are present almost everywhere: in the air, on our skin and hair, in our noses and mouths, in our intestinal tracts, in our food, on kitchen equipment, in garden soil and in water. Some are mobile and can swim around in liquids but most cannot move by themselves. These are only transferred by direct contact.

GROWTH AND MULTIPLICATION

If bacteria are supplied with food, water and a warm temperature, they will grow and reproduce by a process known as binary fission. The bacterial cell grows to a maximum size by absorbing simple substances from its environment and then splits into two new identical cells. In optimum conditions (the very best conditions) for growth (see Chapter 2) bacteria will divide into two approximately every twenty minutes.

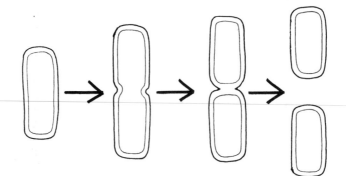

Bacteria reproduce by a process known as binary fission

One bacterium will therefore produce two bacteria after twenty minutes. These two bacteria will then both grow and divide into two after a further twenty minutes making a total of four bacteria after forty minutes. After sixty minutes there will be eight bacteria and after five or six hours there will be thousands of bacteria.

Study the following table to see how quickly the number of bacteria in food can increase. Can you fill in the spaces?

	20 min	40 min	60 min
0 hours	2	4	8
1 hour	16	32	64
2 hours	128	256	
3 hours	1024	2048	4096
4 hours		16 384	
5 hours	65 536		262 144

After six hours in optimum conditions it is possible for one bacterium to become 262 144 bacteria. These bacteria will continue to grow at the same rate until food or an essential growth factor is no longer available or until the presence of poisonous waste products inhibits their growth.

PATHOGENS

Only a few of the thousands of different types of bacteria are responsible for causing illness. Those which do are known as pathogens.
Certain pathogens can make food poisonous by growing and multiplying in it and must normally be present in large numbers in order to
cause illness. Small numbers of most types of pathogenic bacteria can
be swallowed with food without causing any ill effects. However, food
can contain large numbers of food poisoning bacteria and yet look and
smell perfectly wholesome.

SPOILAGE BACTERIA

Certain bacteria are capable of spoiling food without making it
poisonous. The change in odour, taste and appearance of pasteurised
milk on keeping is due to acids produced by bacteria as they grow in
the milk. Spoilage bacteria are not usually pathogenic. However, if food
has been kept in conditions which allow the multiplication of spoilage
bacteria, any food poisoning bacteria which are also present will have
had a chance to multiply.

USEFUL BACTERIA

Many bacteria perform useful functions and are essential for certain
processes, for example:

1. The manufacture of cheese and yoghurt.

2. The production of some antibiotics and some vitamins.

3. The production of manure from decaying vegetable matter.

YEASTS AND MOULDS

Micro-organisms are living things which are individually too small to be
seen without a microscope. There are many different types. The ones
most frequently found in food, apart from bacteria, are yeasts and
moulds.
    Yeasts do not cause food poisoning but some types are capable of
causing food spoilage. They usually spoil acid foods with a high sugar

content, e.g. fruit juices, yoghurts, wines. One type of yeast has great commercial importance because it is used for the production of bread and alcohol (beer, wine and cider).

Moulds do not normally cause food poisoning although some of them can produce mycotoxins (poisonous substances). Moulds present in grain or nuts which are stored in damp conditions produce mycotoxins which may cause cancer. Food is frequently spoiled by moulds, particularly fairly dry or acid food. Black or blue-green moulds are a familiar sight on bread and citrus fruits. Some moulds are used in the production of antibiotics and blue cheeses.

SUMMARY

1. Bacteria are very small; approximately 1 000 000 would cover a pin-head.

2. In optimum conditions for growth, bacteria will divide into two approximately every twenty minutes.

3. There are thousands of different types of bacteria but only a few of them can cause food poisoning.

4. Bacteria, yeasts and moulds are all micro-organisms which are frequently present in food.

Chapter 2

The Growth Requirements of Food Poisoning Bacteria

In order to grow and multiply, bacteria require four things: warmth, food, moisture and time.

WARMTH

The bacteria which cause food poisoning prefer to live at the temperature of the human body, 37 °C (98.6 °F), and it is at this temperature that they will grow and multiply at the fastest rate. As the temperature increases from 37 °C (98.6 °F) to 63 °C (145 °F) the rate of growth slows down and at temperatures above this bacteria will gradually be killed. The length of time and the temperature required to kill them will depend on the type of bacteria and the food involved. They are normally killed in 1–2 minutes in boiling water, unless they are able to form spores (see p. 8).

If the temperature of the food is decreased from 37 °C (98.6 °F) to 10 °C (50 °F) the bacteria will continue to multiply but the rate of multiplication will slow down as the temperature decreases. Bacteria are not killed by low temperatures but they are dormant. This means that they stay alive but stop growing and multiplying. Food poisoning bacteria will not grow at the temperature of the domestic refrigerator, 1–4 °C (34–39 °F), but some spoilage bacteria are able to grow and multiply slowly. When the foods are removed from the refrigerator and warmed up, the rate of bacterial growth increases. Pathogenic and spoilage bacteria remain dormant even in frozen food, but as soon as the food is thawed they will start to grow and multiply again.

In the summer, the temperature in a badly ventilated kitchen can reach 30 °C (86 °F) which is a temperature at which bacteria can multiply very rapidly. For this reason foods should not be allowed to stand for any length of time in a kitchen. Any preparation should be done as quickly as possible and then the food should be stored in a refrigerator until it is ready to be served.

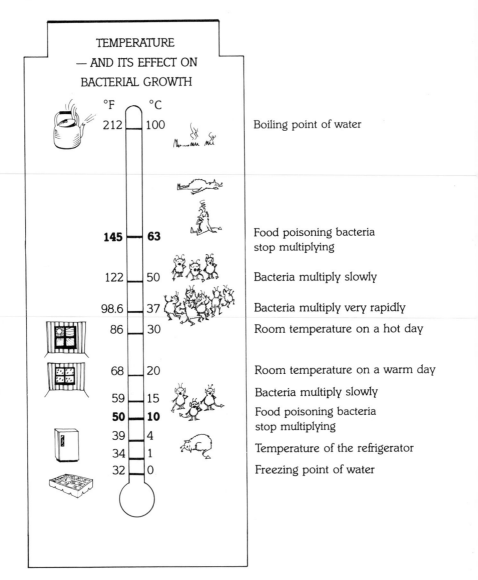

TEMPERATURE
— AND ITS EFFECT ON
BACTERIAL GROWTH

°F	°C	
212	100	Boiling point of water
145	63	Food poisoning bacteria stop multiplying
122	50	Bacteria multiply slowly
98.6	37	Bacteria multiply very rapidly
86	30	Room temperature on a hot day
68	20	Room temperature on a warm day
59	15	Bacteria multiply slowly
50	10	Food poisoning bacteria stop multiplying
39	4	Temperature of the refrigerator
34	1	
32	0	Freezing point of water

FOOD

Like all living things bacteria need food. They will live and multiply in many foodstuffs, particularly those which are high in protein and moisture. The foods that we eat that most frequently support bacterial growth are:

1. Meats, poultry and meat products (meat pies and pasties, sausages).

2. Stocks, gravies, stews and sauces.

3. Milk, cream and egg products (custards, trifles).

The following foods do not normally support the growth of food-poisoning bacteria:

1. Acid foods (pickles, citrus fruits).

2. Foods with a high concentration of salt (salted meats, anchovies, olives).

3. Foods with a high concentration of sugar (jams, syrups).

4. Fatty foods (butter, cooking oils, fatty fish).

5. Dry foods (biscuits, flour).

Although bacteria thrive on foods enjoyed by humans, a crumb lodged in a crack on a table or a smear of blood on an unwashed chopping board is sufficient food for thousands of bacteria.

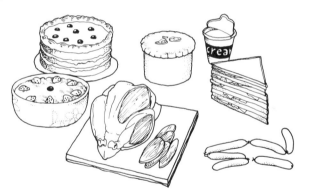

Some of the foods which support bacterial growth

MOISTURE

Like all living things bacteria require moisture for growth. Most foods contain sufficient water for bacterial growth but dehydrated products such as milk powder, dried soup powder and dried egg powder will not allow the growth of bacteria. In dried products bacteria survive but remain dormant until the powders are reconstituted. If a pint of milk is made up from milk powder, it must be stored in a refrigerator as soon as the water is added, to prevent any bacteria present from multiplying.

TIME

If bacteria are provided with food, water and a temperature near 37 °C (98.6 °F), they will divide into two every twenty minutes. A few bacteria cannot cause illness but if food contaminated with bacteria is kept for a sufficiently long time in the right conditions the number of bacteria will increase, making the food poisonous. If food is eaten shortly after it is cooked or prepared, the risk of food poisoning is considerably reduced.

AEROBES AND ANAEROBES

Bacteria differ from one another in their requirements for air. Most of them require the presence of air to grow and multiply and these are called aerobes. Some do not require the presence of air to grow and multiply and these are called anaerobes.

SPORES

When bacteria are growing and multiplying we say they are in the vegetative state. In this state they are fairly easily destroyed by heat or chemicals. Some bacteria, but not all, can exist in another form — the spore form. A spore is a rounded body which forms inside the bacterial cell when conditions become unfavourable for growth or multiplication. The rest of the cell then gradually disintegrates leaving only the spore. This spore can resist very high temperatures and high concentrations of chemicals that would kill bacteria in the vegetative state. They can survive at least four hours in boiling water and so they are not destroyed by normal cooking methods. Spores are also formed when there is insufficient moisture present. They can survive for years without food or water, but when conditions again become favourable the spores return to the vegetative state and continue to grow and multiply.

SUMMARY

1. The four requirements for bacterial growth are warmth, food, moisture and time.

2. The bacteria which cause food-poisoning grow best at 37 °C (98.6 °F).

3. The temperature and humidity of the kitchen provide excellent conditions for the growth and multiplication of bacteria.

4. Bacteria are not killed by the cold but those which cause food-poisoning stop multiplying in a refrigerator.

5. Bacteria grow best in foods which are high in moisture and are not too acid, not too sugary and not too salty.

6. Bacteria cannot grow and multiply without moisture but they can remain dormant in dried foods.

7. Bacteria in the vegetative state are killed after two minutes in boiling water.

8. Some bacteria form spores which are only destroyed after several hours in boiling water.

Chapter 3

What is Food Poisoning?

Food poisoning is an illness brought about by eating harmful food. The symptoms are usually vomiting, diarrhoea and abdominal pains. Vomiting and diarrhoea are the body's method of disposing of harmful substances from the digestive tract thus preventing them from getting into the blood stream. In a few types of food poisoning the poisons enter the blood stream, causing illness in the body generally, with a wide variety of symptoms.

CAUSES OF FOOD POISONING

The causes of food poisoning fall into four main categories.

1.   *Bacterial food poisoning*   The vast majority of all food poisoning cases are caused by bacteria. The food is poisonous because it has been contaminated by pathogenic bacteria which have been allowed to multiply during incorrect storage of the food.

2.   *Viral food poisoning*   Certain viruses which cause vomiting and diarrhoea can be transmitted by water and food. Viruses require living tissue for growth and therefore will not multiply in the food. The food is merely a means of transport into the human body. They are destroyed by the temperatures reached in normal cooking methods and so viral food poisoning is usually transmitted by food which has not been cooked or has been handled after cooking by a human who is a carrier of the virus. Inadequately cooked shellfish collected from sewage-contaminated waters have caused viral food poisoning.

3.   *Chemical food poisoning*   The food is poisonous because it has been contaminated by chemicals during the growth, preparation, storage or cooking of the food. Most cases of chemical food poisoning are caused by carelessness in the home or an industrial establishment. Pesticides, paraffin, detergents and sterilising agents should be stored away from food and in such a way that they will not spill or leak from their containers. There are strict regulations for food producers and food manufacturers governing the use of insecticidal sprays, pesticides, food additives and packaging materials. There have been a few

outbreaks of zinc poisoning due to the use of galvanised equipment with acid foods. Chipped enamel vessels can cause antimony poisoning, particularly if used with acid foods.

4. *Vegetable food poisoning* Certain plants naturally contain substances which are poisonous to human beings, for example toadstools, hemlock, deadly nightshade, rhubarb leaves. The most common cause of vegetable food poisoning is the toadstool which can easily be mistaken for a mushroom. The consumption of raw or undercooked red kidney beans is also a cause of severe vomiting.

BACTERIAL FOOD POISONING

How many bacteria must be present to cause illness?

Quite frequently we eat food which contains a few food poisoning bacteria but small numbers of bacteria do not cause illness. Approximately one million bacteria must be present before a healthy adult will feel any harmful effects. If approximately one tenth this number are present, a child under one year, an old person or a sick person would be affected. Special care must therefore be taken when preparing food for people in these categories.

Food poisoning is occasionally fatal. The deaths caused by food poisoning are usually in very young babies or in old or severely ill people.

Incubation period

This is the time that passes between the entry of the poisonous food into the body and the occurrence of the first symptoms. The length of the incubation period helps to decide which type of bacteria has caused the food poisoning. Some types of bacteria cause food poisoning with a relatively long incubation period (up to 2 days) and other types of bacteria cause food poisoning with a relatively short incubation period (2 hours). The length of the incubation period also depends on the number of bacteria present as well as the type of bacteria causing the food poisoning. If the food is very heavily contaminated with a certain type of bacteria, the incubation period will be shorter than if the food is contaminated with only half the number of the same type of bacteria.

Duration

The duration of the illness is the time between the appearance of the first symptoms of food poisoning and the clearing up of the last ones. When all the symptoms of food poisoning have gone, it does not necessarily mean that there are no harmful bacteria in the intestinal tract but that the numbers present are no longer sufficient to produce symptoms(see convalescent carriers p. 14).

THE BACTERIA WHICH CAUSE FOOD POISONING

The following bacteria are known to cause food poisoning:

Salmonella
Staphylococcus aureus
Clostridium perfringens
Clostridium botulinum
Bacillus cereus

All bacteria have two names:

The generic name which is written first and with a capital letter (equivalent to our surname), e.g. *Clostridium, Bacillus. The specific name* which is written with a small letter after the generic name (equivalent to our first names, e.g. *perfringens, cereus.*

There are approximately 2000 species of the *Salmonella* genus (e.g. *Salmonella typhimurium, Salmonella hadar, Salmonella newport*) but since most of them cause food poisoning it is usual to talk about *Salmonella* food poisoning without distinguishing which species is actually the cause.   *Salmonella, Staphylococcus aureus, Clostridium perfringens* and *Bacillus cereus* are all common causes of food poisoning in the UK and many other countries. It is important to know how these particular bacteria normally gain access to food and what measures can be taken to avoid this or to prevent their multiplication.

Several other bacteria can cause food poisoning but do so far less frequently than those mentioned above (see Appendix 1).

Food poisoning caused by *Clostridium botulinum* is extremely rare but it is so severe that extra precautions must be taken to prevent its occurrence.

SUMMARY

1. The symptoms of food poisoning are usually vomiting, diarrhoea and abdominal pains.

2. The four main types of food poisoning are:
   (a) Bacterial food poisoning — the most common.
   (b) Viral food poisoning.
   (c) Chemical food poisoning.
   (d) Vegetable food poisoning.

3. The incubation period and the duration of bacterial food poisoning give an indication of the type of bacteria which has caused the illness.

4. *Salmonella, Staphylococcus aureus, Clostridium perfringens* and *Bacillus cereus* frequently cause food poisoning in Britain and many other countries.

Chapter 4

Pathogenic Bacteria

HOW PATHOGENIC BACTERIA GAIN ACCESS TO THE KITCHEN

1. Raw meat

Animals and poultry frequently carry pathogenic bacteria in their intestines. When the animals are slaughtered and dressed, these bacteria may spread over the surface of the meat where they will grow and multiply rapidly unless the meat is refrigerated immediately and kept under refrigeration during transport and storage in the butcher's shop. If these storage rules are observed the bacteria on contaminated meat will remain dormant, but they will be able to grow and multiply again as soon as the meat is removed from refrigerated storage into normal room temperatures. However reputable the supplier, raw meat often carries small numbers of pathogenic bacteria. These will normally be killed in the cooking process, but care must be taken by the food handler not to let them have a chance to multiply and not to let them spread to foods which have already been cooked. (See cross-contamination, p. 15.)

2. Food handlers

Pathogenic bacteria from food handlers can be spread into food, usually via the hands, during preparation and service. Everybody carries bacteria in their mouth, nose, intestine and on their skin and some of these bacteria will inevitably be transferred to food.

Carriers   A small percentage of the population are carriers of pathogenic bacteria and although they do not have the symptoms of food poisoning, pathogenic bacteria are present in their intestines and are therefore passed in their faeces. There are two types of carrier:

(a) *Convalescent carriers*   People who have recently had food poisoning and who although perfectly fit again continue to pass small numbers of pathogenic bacteria in their faeces.

(b) *Healthy carriers*   People who have not suffered the symptoms

14

of food poisoning but nevertheless are carrying pathogenic bacteria in their intestines.

Convalescent and healthy carriers run a high risk of contaminating their hands with food poisoning bacteria on visiting the WC. Convalescent carriers will know the risk they are running and should if possible be given work which does not involve the handling of food until they have stopped excreting pathogenic bacteria. Where this is not possible, e.g. at home, extra attention must be paid to the thorough washing of hands and scrubbing of nails.

3. Animals and insects

Flies, rats, mice, birds, other insects and animals including pets frequently carry pathogenic bacteria in their intestines and on their feet and fur and must therefore not be allowed to come into contact with food or equipment which will be used for food preparation.

4. Dust

Soil contains spores of some of the pathogenic bacteria. Raw vegetables must therefore always be cleaned thoroughly in a section of the kitchen used only for this purpose and then transferred to another section for further preparation.

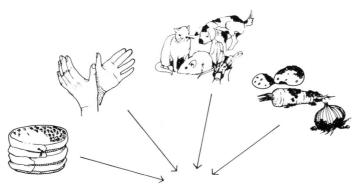

All these carry food poisoning bacteria

CROSS-CONTAMINATION

Cross-contamination is the transfer of bacteria from a contaminated source to an uncontaminated food (usually freshly cooked food). If this food is suitable for bacterial growth and is left for some time in a warm room, the few bacteria which have been transferred to it will multiply to large numbers and when the food is eventually eaten it will cause food poisoning. If the original contaminated source was a raw food, it will not usually be a cause of food poisoning because the bacteria present are later destroyed by cooking.

Causes of cross-contamination   Bacteria can be transferred from a contaminated source to an uncontaminated food by:

(a) Using a chopping board, a working surface or other kitchen equipment for the preparation of two different foods without washing it thoroughly between each use.

(b) Using a knife or other utensil without washing it thoroughly between each use.

(c) The hands of a food handler which are not washed in between preparing different types of food, e.g. raw and cooked meat, or after touching any source of bacteria, e.g. the nose, mouth, hair, pets.

(d) Incorrect positioning of foods in a refrigerator. For example, raw meat must always be placed below cooked food so that blood (which often contains pathogenic bacteria) cannot drip on to the cooked food.

Examples of cross-contamination

1. *A mincer which has been used for raw meat and then for cooked corned beef.*
   A chef working in a busy kitchen is making liver pâté. He minces the raw liver and decides to leave cleaning the mincer until he has got the pâté into the oven.

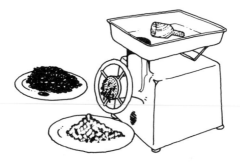

Before the first chef has finished the preparation of the pâté, a second chef uses the mincer for some corned beef which is to be used for a rissole. In this way, some bacteria from the liver are transferred to the corned beef.

The rissoles are left in the kitchen for several hours before they are cooked. During this time the bacteria increase to a sufficient number to cause food poisoning. As all the ingredients in the rissoles have already been cooked, they are only lightly browned before serving and the temperature reached in the centre of the rissoles during cooking is not sufficiently high to kill all the bacteria.

How food poisoning could have been prevented: By thoroughly washing the mincer immediately after use.

2. *A knife which has been used for cutting raw meat and not washed thoroughly before it is used for slicing cooked meat.*

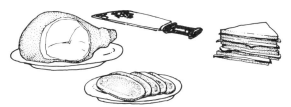

A chef is preparing sandwiches for a children's picnic. He has just finished cutting up raw meat for a casserole and as he is in a hurry he gives his knife a quick wipe on his overall and continues to use it to slice some ham.

A smear of blood from the raw meat is left on the knife and when the cooked ham is sliced with the same knife a few pathogenic bacteria are transferred to it. The ham is then used to make sandwiches.

It is a warm day and before the sandwiches are eaten the bacteria increase to sufficient numbers to cause food poisoning.

How food poisoning could have been prevented: By washing the knife with detergent and rinsing in very hot water after using it for raw meat and before using it for cooked meat.

3. *A chef develops a heavy cold but does not report it to his employer and continues to work as usual on the preparation of desserts.*

While piping cream on to a trifle the chef sneezes. He naturally turns away from the food and sneezes into his handkerchief but he does not wash his hands before continuing with his work. A few bacteria from the handkerchief are transferred to his hands and from there to the cream on the trifle. The trifle is put on the sweet trolley and most of it is eaten fairly quickly but two portions remain for several hours in the warm dining room. Those who ate the trifle at the beginning of the evening did not develop food poisoning but by the time the final two portions were eaten the bacteria had increased to a sufficient number to cause illness.

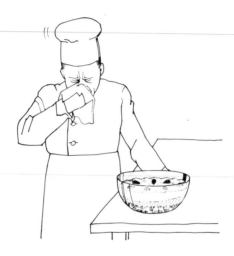

How food poisoning could have been prevented: By washing his hands after touching the handkerchief. It is preferable to use disposable paper handkerchiefs which are destroyed after one use.

4. *Uncooked steak is placed on the top shelf of the refrigerator and uncovered roast chicken on the bottom shelf.*

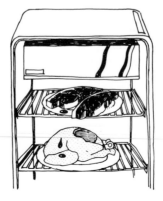

A drop of blood from the uncooked steak drips on to the uncovered roast chicken stored below it.

A few pathogenic bacteria in the drop of blood are transferred to the chicken. They do not multiply in the refrigerator but remain dormant.

The chicken is served at a buffet on a warm afternoon. It is on display for three hours before it is eaten and during this time the bacteria increase to sufficient numbers to cause food poisoning.

How food poisoning could have been prevented: By using different refrigerators for storing raw and cooked meat or by placing the uncooked steak at the bottom of the refrigerator and the cooked chicken at the top.

SUMMARY

1. The main sources of pathogenic bacteria in the kitchen are raw meat, food handlers, animals, insects and dust.

2. Cross-contamination is the transfer of bacteria from a contaminated source to uncontaminated food.

Chapter 5

Salmonella

Salmonella is a short, thin, rod-shaped bacterium.

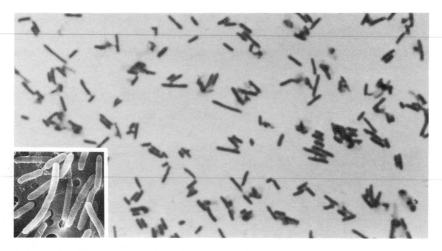

Salmonella   Main photograph, light micrograph × 1400
Inset, scanning electron micrograph × 2860

More outbreaks of food poisoning in the UK are caused by *Salmonella* than by any other bacteria.

People can be severely ill with *Salmonella* food poisoning and there are between twenty and fifty fatal cases each year, usually in elderly, very young or sick people.

TYPE OF FOOD POISONING

Salmonella causes infective food poisoning.

Large numbers of living bacteria must be present in the food when it is eaten. Some of them will be destroyed by the acid in the stomach but some will be protected by food and pass through to the small intestine where the near neutral conditions allow them to multiply. As they increase in numbers, some of the cells die and release a poisonous substance which causes fever, diarrhoea and vomiting. Since it takes some time for the bacteria to increase in numbers to a level which causes symptoms, the incubation period is relatively long.

Incubation period   12–36 hours
Duration of illness   1–8 days
Symptoms   Fever, headache, abdominal pains, diarrhoea
                      and vomiting

NATURAL ORIGIN OF *SALMONELLA*

1. *Salmonella* is commonly found in animal fodder and is therefore found in the intestines of many farm animals, particularly poultry.

2. Mice, rats, domestic pets, flies and birds also often carry *Salmonella* in their intestines and on their fur and feet.

MEANS OF ACCESS TO FOOD

1. Brought into the kitchen on or in foods of animal origin, e.g. poultry, meat, unpasteurised milk, dried egg powder.

   Salmonella is normally present only on the surface of raw meat but is often present in the central cavity of poultry or in the centre of minced meat products such as sausages and hamburgers. These foods may cause poisoning if they are inadequately cooked or they may contaminate other foods which have already been cooked.

   Unpasteurised milk is sometimes contaminated with *Salmonella*. Pasteurisation destroys *Salmonella*.

   Duck eggs frequently harbour *Salmonella* and it has recently been found that some hen eggs do but it is thought to be only a small proportion. The shell of both types may be contaminated with *Salmonella*.

2. Insects, birds, vermin and domestic pets can spread *Salmonella* into food if they are allowed to be present in the kitchen.

3. People working in the kitchen are sometimes, unknown to them, carrying *Salmonella* in their intestines and may contaminate food if hands are not washed after a visit to the WC.

DESTRUCTION

Salmonella is readily killed by heat. It does not form a spore.

FOODS USUALLY INVOLVED

Foods causing this type of food poisoning have either been cooked inadequately or have been contaminated after cooking, e.g. poultry which has not been properly defrosted, cold meats which have been cross-contaminated.

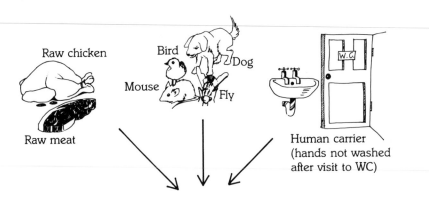

Raw chicken

Raw meat

Bird

Dog

Mouse

Fly

Human carrier
(hands not washed
after visit to WC)

Any of these may contaminate the foods below with *Salmonella*

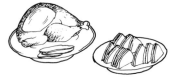

These foods are not cooked again

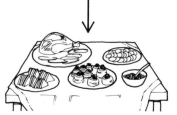

They are kept warm for several hours

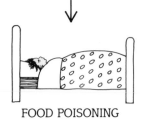

FOOD POISONING

PREVENTIVE MEASURES

1. Thaw frozen food completely before cooking. When thawing poultry always follow the instructions on the wrapper. A 30 lb turkey would take approximately 48 hours to thaw in a refrigerator.

2. Cook food thoroughly making sure the temperature at the centre of the food is high enough to kill bacteria.

3. Use different surfaces and equipment e.g. chopping boards, knives, etc. for preparing raw food and cooked food.

4. Clean all equipment thoroughly after each use.

5. Store raw and cooked foods (particularly meat) separately.

6. Wash hands after handling raw meat and poultry.

7. Keep food as cold as possible to prevent multiplication of *Salmonella*.

A TYPICAL CHAIN OF EVENTS LEADING TO FOOD POISONING BY *SALMONELLA*

Roast chicken is a favourite on the menu at a restaurant where many people have their midday meal. Normally the chickens are taken from the deep freeze the previous evening and left to defrost in the refrigerator overnight.

One evening the chef forgot to remove the chickens from the deep freeze so he arrived at work early the next morning and put them in a sink of hot water for two hours. He then ran some hot water inside the chicken carcasses and managed to melt some of the ice. He hastily stuffs the chickens and puts them into the oven to cook for lunchtime thinking that the rest of the ice will melt in the heat of the oven.

After the normal cooking time he is relieved to find that the flesh appears to be perfectly cooked and so he serves it at lunchtime as usual with a portion of stuffing.

The following day several people in the area have to go to their doctors with severe headaches, abdominal pains, diarrhoea and vomiting. They are questioned about where they had eaten their meals during the last 36 hours and an outbreak of *Salmonella* food poisoning is traced to the restaurant where the chickens were served.

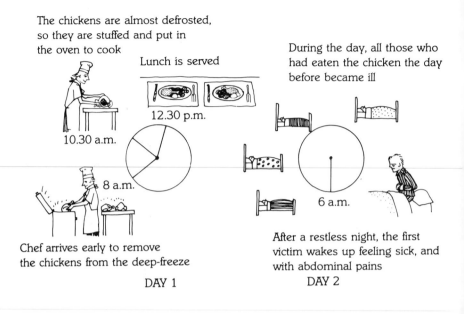

The chickens are almost defrosted, so they are stuffed and put in the oven to cook

Lunch is served

12.30 p.m.

10.30 a.m.

8 a.m.

During the day, all those who had eaten the chicken the day before became ill

6 a.m.

Chef arrives early to remove the chickens from the deep-freeze

DAY 1

After a restless night, the first victim wakes up feeling sick, and with abdominal pains

DAY 2

Fault

Frozen meat, particularly poultry, must be thawed completely before commencing cooking. If ice is present in the centre of the chicken, a great deal of heat is used to melt it. It will take far longer for the internal temperature to equal the external temperature than it would if the chicken were completely defrosted. Even if the chicken is cooked for the recommended time, the temperature in the centre of the bird at the end of the cooking time is not sufficiently high to kill *Salmonella* but is probably an optimum temperature for its multiplication. It is advisable to cook stuffing separately and not in the bird, where it will slow down heat penetration.

Chapter 6

Staphylococcus aureus

Staphylococcus aureus is a round bacterium.

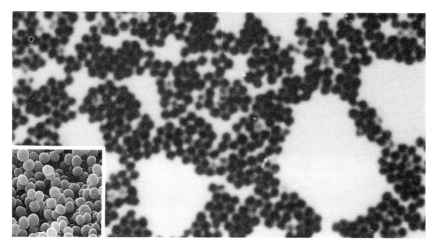

S. *aureus*   Main photograph, light micrograph × 3300
Inset, scanning electron micrograph × 3945

The symptoms of food poisoning caused by *Staphylococcus aureus* are severe for a short period of time but the illness is rarely fatal.

TYPE OF FOOD POISONING

Staphylococcus aureus causes toxic food poisoning. Whilst growing and multiplying in food stored at a warm temperature, it produces a toxin (a poisonous substance). When the food is swallowed the toxin irritates the stomach lining causing vomiting. The incubation period is therefore relatively short and the main symptom is vomiting.

Incubation period	1–7 hours
Duration of illness	6–24 hours
Symptoms	Vomiting, sometimes abdominal pains and diarrhoea

NATURAL ORIGIN OF *STAPHYLOCOCCUS AUREUS*

Staphylococcus aureus is frequently present in the human nose and throat and on the skin of healthy people. It is known as a commensal because it is completely harmless when present in these areas. It is found also in large numbers in boils, styes and septic cuts.

Staphylococcus aureus is sometimes present in unpasteurised milk.

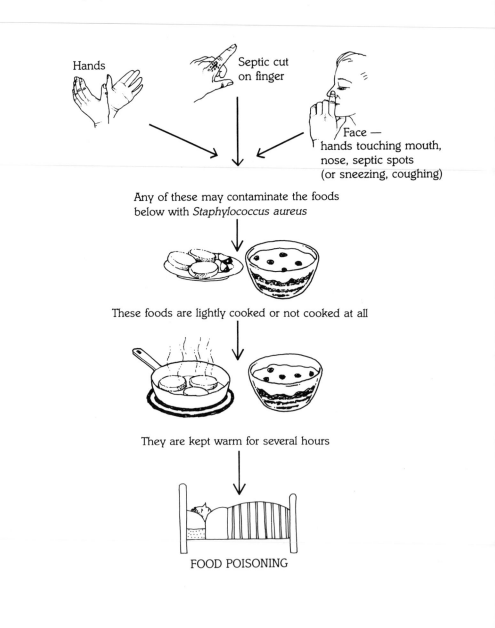

Hands

Septic cut on finger

Face — hands touching mouth, nose, septic spots (or sneezing, coughing)

Any of these may contaminate the foods below with *Staphylococcus aureus*

These foods are lightly cooked or not cooked at all

They are kept warm for several hours

FOOD POISONING

MEANS OF ACCESS TO FOOD

1. People working in the kitchen who sneeze or cough over food or who have septic cuts, boils, styes, etc. and do not cover them with an adequate waterproof dressing.

2. Unpasteurised milk and products made from unpasteurised milk which are not cooked or only lightly cooked.

DESTRUCTION

Staphylococcus aureus does not form a spore and is therefore readily killed by heat (1–2 minutes in boiling water) BUT the toxin which it produces in food is more resistant to heat than the bacterial cell and can withstand up to 30 minutes in boiling water. It is therefore possible for lightly cooked food to contain active toxin but no live bacteria. This food will still cause food poisoning.

FOODS USUALLY INVOLVED

Foods causing *Staphylococcus aureus* food poisoning are usually those which have been contaminated by the food handler after they have been cooked and are then eaten cold or after a mild reheating process, e.g. sliced cold meats, cream dishes, custards and other milk products and stuffed rolled joints which have not been cooked through to the centre. *Staphylococcus* is able to grow in higher concentrations of salt than the other food poisoning bacteria and therefore outbreaks involving salty foods, e.g. ham, are often traced to *Staphylococcus*.

PREVENTIVE MEASURES

1. Maintain a high standard of personal hygiene.

2. Handle food as little as possible. Always use serving tongs for food which will not be heated again.

3. Keep food as cold as possible to prevent the multiplication of *Staphylococcus aureus*.

A TYPICAL CHAIN OF EVENTS LEADING TO FOOD POISONING BY *STAPHYLOCOCCUS AUREUS*

At a school canteen, custard is served most days with the pudding. As it is fairly easy to prepare, a new member of staff was allocated this task. He starts work at 8.00 a.m. and on one particular morning as there is no other urgent work, he starts by preparing the custard. At 8.30 a.m. he moves on to another task and leaves the custard to cool but suddenly wonders if he remembered to add the sugar. He tastes it with a spoon and thinks it seems sweet enough but just checks it again using the same spoon without washing it. He is then quite satisfied that the sugar has been added. The custard is left in the kitchen for the rest of the morning and at 12.15 p.m. it is warmed up and served for lunch at 12.30 p.m.

That afternoon several children start to feel sick and have acute stomach pains. By 5.30 p.m. that evening all the children who had eaten the custard are ill and an outbreak of food poisoning caused by *Staphylococcus aureus* is confirmed.

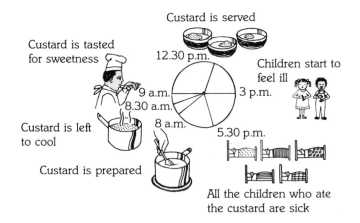

Custard is served

Custard is tasted for sweetness

Children start to feel ill

Custard is left to cool

Custard is prepared

All the children who ate the custard are sick

Fault

A spoon which has been put into the mouth must never be returned to food without first washing it. *Staphylococcus aureus* may be transferred from the mouth to food via the spoon. If the food is left for some time at a warm temperature the bacteria will grow, multiply and produce toxins. If the food is only lightly reheated the toxins will not be destroyed.

Chapter 7

Clostridium perfringens

previously known as
Clostridium welchii *is not killed by cooking*

Clostridium perfringens is a rod-shaped bacterium. It can form a spore when conditions are unfavourable for growth and is also an anaerobe so grows best in the absence of oxygen.

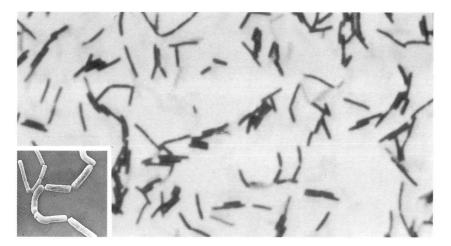

Cl. perfringens Main photograph, light micrograph × 1400
Inset, scanning electron micrograph × 4100

Clostridium perfringens is the second most common cause of food poisoning in the UK. There have been a few fatal cases in elderly or sick people.

TYPE OF FOOD POISONING

Clostridium perfringens does not produce toxin when it is multiplying in food stored at a warm temperature, but when that food is eaten the bacteria form spores and at the same time a toxin, which irritates the intestinal wall causing diarrhoea. This is not exactly the same as toxic food poisoning or infective food poisoning but has some characteristics of both. The incubation period is longer than with toxic food poisoning

29

as caused by *Staphylococcus aureus* and shorter than infective food poisoning as caused by *Salmonella*.

Incubation period	8–22 hours
Duration of illness	12–24 hours
Symptoms	Abdominal pains and diarrhoea. The patient rarely vomits.

NATURAL ORIGIN OF *CLOSTRIDIUM PERFRINGENS*

1. *Cl. perfringens* is frequently present in human and animal intestines.

2. Flies and bluebottles are usually heavily infected with *Cl. perfringens*.

3. Spores of *Cl. perfringens* are found in soil.

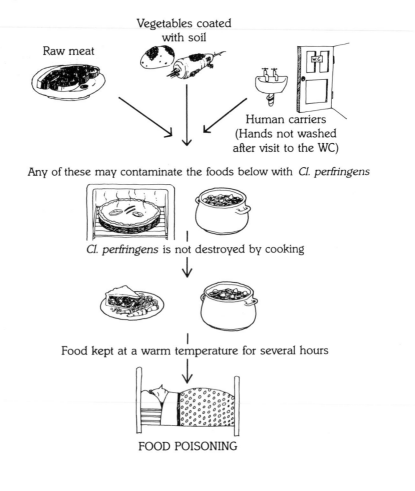

Vegetables coated with soil

Raw meat

Human carriers
(Hands not washed after visit to the WC)

Any of these may contaminate the foods below with *Cl. perfringens*

Cl. perfringens is not destroyed by cooking

Food kept at a warm temperature for several hours

FOOD POISONING

MEANS OF ACCESS TO FOOD

1. Brought into the kitchen on raw meat. The meat itself may cause food poisoning since *Cl. perfringens* can survive cooking processes by forming a spore. Bacteria from the raw meat may also be transferred to cooked foods in careless preparation.

2. Vegetables coated with soil or dust from sacks or packing cases may contaminate foods with *Cl. perfringens* if the soil or dust settles on food.

3. People working in the kitchen may be carrying *Cl. perfringens* in their intestines and may spread the bacteria into food if their hands are not washed after a visit to the WC.

DESTRUCTION

The spores of *Cl. perfringens* are not destroyed by normal cooking methods. They can withstand boiling, steaming, stewing or braising for up to 4 hours. The spores do not multiply but if the food is cooled slowly or kept warm (between 10 °C (50 °F) and 63 °C (145 °F)) for some time before serving, the spores germinate producing vegetative bacteria which multiply rapidly at these temperatures.

FOODS USUALLY INVOLVED

As it does not grow readily in the presence of oxygen, *Cl. perfringens* is most frequently found reproducing rapidly at the bottom of a lukewarm meat casserole or stock pot or at the centre of large food masses where there is little air (oxygen), e.g. meat pies, minced meat dishes. Reheated meat dishes are also frequently a cause of *Cl. perfringens* food poisoning since the spore it forms will survive each reheating process.

Most outbreaks involve a large number of people because *Cl. perfringens* is more commonly found in foods that have been prepared in bulk.

PREVENTIVE MEASURES

1. Use separate preparation areas for raw food (especially meat and vegetables) and cooked food.

2. Cool cooked foods rapidly and refrigerate promptly. To do this it may be necessary to break up large volumes of meat and cool and store it in separate smaller containers. Large joints of meat should be removed from the cooking liquor immediately after cooking to speed up cooling.

3. Use different surfaces and equipment e.g. chopping boards, knives, etc. for preparing raw food and cooked food.

4. Clean all equipment thoroughly after each use.

5. Store raw foods (particularly meat and unwashed vegetables) away from cooked food.

6. Wash hands after handling raw meat and unwashed vegetables.

7. If reheating of food is necessary, it must be reheated rapidly and thoroughly and then served quickly. Never reheat meat products more than once.

A TYPICAL CHAIN OF EVENTS LEADING TO FOOD POISONING BY *CLOSTRIDIUM PERFRINGENS*

The staff in a works canteen are responsible for preparing a main meal for all the people at the factory. There are two shifts. The early shift eats lunch at 11.00 a.m. The late shift eats at 2.00 p.m.

One day, one of the dishes on the menu is beef casserole. The chef preparing the casserole gathers together the ingredients (beef, onions, carrots and swedes) and takes them to the working surface where he usually does his preparation. He cuts the beef and puts it on one side and then scrapes the vegetables, chops them and puts everything together in the casserole which is then cooked in time for the first shift. It is taken from the oven a few minutes before 11.00 a.m. and served piping hot to the people on the first shift. However, not all of it is used so rather than see it wasted the staff decide to leave it in the warming cabinet to keep it warm for the second shift. The temperature in the warming cabinet is 45 °C (113 °F).

That night some of the people from the factory start to feel ill with severe abdominal pains and diarrhoea. An outbreak of food poisoning caused by *Cl. perfringens* is confirmed and traced to the beef casserole although it is only the people on the second shift who are ill and none of those from the first shift are affected.

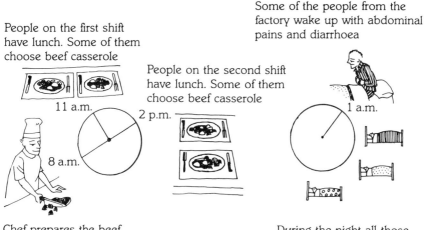

People on the first shift have lunch. Some of them choose beef casserole

11 a.m.

8 a.m.

Chef prepares the beef casserole and puts it in the oven to cook

DAY 1

People on the second shift have lunch. Some of them choose beef casserole

2 p.m.

Some of the people from the factory wake up with abdominal pains and diarrhoea

1 a.m.

During the night all those from the second shift who ate beef casserole are ill

DAY 2

Faults

1. Separate working areas, equipment and utensils should be used for preparing raw meat and vegetables.

2. Foods which are suitable for bacterial growth should never be kept warm. If they are not served immediately they must be kept hot, at a temperature above 63 °C (145 °F) or cold, at a temperature below 10 °C (50 °F). In this case the casserole was kept warm for three hours in between servings. *Cl. perfringens* from either the raw meat or from soil on the vegetables had survived the cooking process by forming spores which were able to germinate, grow and multiply rapidly when the casserole was kept at a temperature of 45 °C (113 °F).

Chapter 8

Clostridium botulinum

Clostridium botulinum has some similar characteristics to *Cl. perfringens.* It is a rod-shaped bacterium and can form a spore when conditions become unfavourable for growth. It is also an anaerobe.

Food poisoning by *Cl. botulinum* is very rare but at the same time it is greatly feared because the majority of cases in the UK are fatal. Life can be saved by giving antitoxin very soon after the onset of the illness.

TYPE OF FOOD POISONING

Clostridium botulinum causes toxic food poisoning. The toxin is produced by the bacteria when they are growing in food under strictly anaerobic conditions (a complete absence of oxygen), e.g. in canned food. The toxin is a highly poisonous substance and people have died after eating only a mouthful of infected food.

Incubation period	2 hours–8 days (usually 12–36 hours)
Duration of illness	Death within a few days unless antitoxin is given to the patient soon after the onset of illness in which case recovery will take place slowly.
Symptoms	Giddiness, double vision, headache, nausea and vomiting. The central nervous system is affected and paralysis of the respiratory tract is the usual cause of death.

NATURAL ORIGIN OF *CLOSTRIDIUM BOTULINUM*

Clostridium botulinum is found in soil and therefore on vegetables. It is also found in fish caught in some areas, notably the waters around Japan.

MEANS OF ACCESS TO FOOD

Clostridium botulinum may be present in the spore form in fish or in the soil on vegetables but does not multiply there in the presence of oxygen. However, if the spore is transferred to an anaerobic, warm and moist environment it will germinate and produce toxin.

DESTRUCTION

Clostridium botulinum can produce a spore which will survive ordinary cooking methods but the toxin produced by it is not heat resistant and will usually be destroyed by boiling for a few minutes.

FOODS USUALLY INVOLVED

Most cases of botulism (food poisoning caused by *Cl. botulinum*) have occurred after eating under-sterilised canned food or food in faulty cans which has been contaminated after sterilisation. Food manufacturers take great care that all *Cl. botulinum* spores are destroyed in processing and only very rarely have commercially canned foods been the cause of this type of food poisoning. In the United States of America, some people can their own vegetables and this has sometimes caused botulism. A Japanese delicacy, of raw fermented fish, has also caused outbreaks of botulism.

PREVENTIVE MEASURES

1. Reject any cans that are blown (if gas has been produced inside the can the contents have probably been under-sterilised and could possibly contain *Cl. botulinum*).

2. Avoid eating home–canned foods.

3. Avoid eating raw fermented fish.

Chapter 9

Bacillus cereus

Bacillus cereus is a rod-shaped bacterium. It can form a spore when conditions are unfavourable for growth. It is an aerobe and therefore requires oxygen for growth.

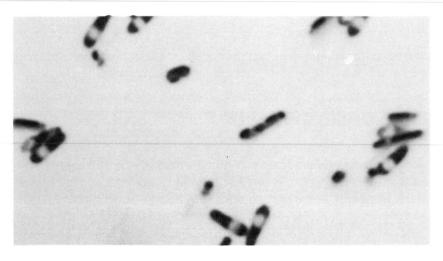

B. cereus   Light micrograph × 1400

The onset of symptoms of *Bacillus cereus* food poisoning can be very sudden but it is usually over fairly quickly. It is most unlikely to be fatal.

TYPE OF FOOD POISONING

Bacillus cereus usually causes toxic food poisoning. Whilst *B. cereus* is growing and multiplying in food stored at a warm temperature, it produces a toxin. When the food is swallowed the toxin irritates the stomach lining causing vomiting.

Incubation period	1–5 hours
Duration	6–24 hours
Symptoms	Vomiting, abdominal pains, occasionally diarrhoea

36

There is a second type of *B. cereus* food poisoning which is rare in the United Kingdom. Toxins are produced in the intestine but not in the food before it is eaten. The incubation period is longer and the main symptom is diarrhoea.

NATURAL ORIGIN OF *BACILLUS CEREUS*

Bacillus cereus is found in the soil and in dust.

MEANS OF ACCESS TO FOOD

The spores of *B. cereus* are brought into the kitchen on cereals, particularly rice. Cornflour and spices are also often contaminated.

DESTRUCTION

The spores of *B. cereus* are not easily destroyed by heat and will survive most cooking processes. They do not multiply but if the food is cooled slowly or kept warm (between 10 °C (50 °F) and 63 °C (145 °F)) for some time before serving, they will germinate producing vegetative bacteria which multiply rapidly at these temperatures and produce a very heat-resistant toxin. If the food is subsequently reheated quickly, the heat is unlikely to be sufficient to destroy the toxin.

FOODS USUALLY INVOLVED

Reheated rice is almost always the cause of *B. cereus* food poisoning.

PREVENTIVE MEASURES

1. Cool cooked food rapidly and refrigerate promptly.
2. If reheating of the food is necessary, it must be reheated rapidly and thoroughly and then served quickly. Never reheat rice more than once.

A TYPICAL CHAIN OF EVENTS LEADING TO FOOD POISONING BY *B. CEREUS*

A housewife has invited twelve friends for a buffet supper party after a visit to the theatre. She has planned to cook a curry and serve it with plain boiled rice. She knows she will not have time to prepare the curry on the evening of the party so she prepares it on the previous evening and after cooking it she cools it quickly and puts it in the refrigerator to store overnight. She also cooks the rice the night before but as there is no room in the refrigerator she covers it and leaves it on the working surface in the kitchen thinking that rice is a 'safe' food anyway.

The next evening, just before the guests arrive, she reheats the curry thoroughly and then warms the rice through over a pan of boiling water and serves both to the guests.

Even before the party is over, several of the guests suddenly start to feel very sick and the others all gradually become ill during the night. An outbreak of food poisoning due to B. cereus is traced to the rice.

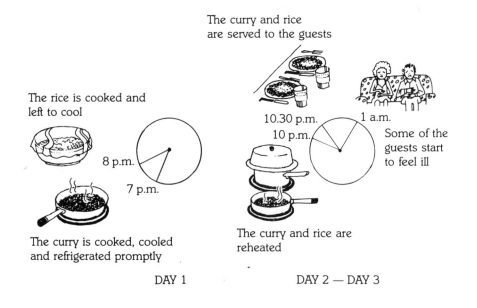

The curry and rice are served to the guests

The rice is cooked and left to cool

8 p.m.

7 p.m.

The curry is cooked, cooled and refrigerated promptly

DAY 1

10.30 p.m.
10 p.m.

1 a.m.
Some of the guests start to feel ill

The curry and rice are reheated

DAY 2 — DAY 3

Fault

Bacteria which had survived the first cooking of the rice by forming spores had germinated into vegetative bacteria, multiplied and produced toxin during long slow cooling overnight. The rice was not reheated sufficiently to destroy the toxin in it.

THE BACTERIA WHICH COMMONLY CAUSE FOOD POISONING

	Salmonella	Staphylococcus	Cl. perfringens	B. cereus
Incuba-tion period	12–36 hours	1–7 hours	8–22 hours	1–5 hours
Duration of illness	1–8 days	6–24 hours	12–24 hours	6–24 hours
Means of access to the kitchen	Poultry and other raw meat. Animals. Human carriers	Mainly through humans, from the nose, mouth, infected wounds and sores	Raw meat. Unwashed vegetables. Human carriers	Cereals especially rice
Foods usually involved	Meat and meat products	Almost any food which has been handled and not cooked or only lightly cooked afterwards, e.g. sliced cold meats, cream and milk products	Meat dishes, e.g. stews, pies, gravy, meat stock. Unwashed vegetables.	Rice
Destruc-tion	Vegetative bac-teria readily destroyed by heat. Does not form spores. Does not pro-duce a toxin	Vegetative bac-teria readily destroyed by heat. Does not form spores. Toxin destroyed by boiling for 30 mins	Forms spores which can survive several hours in boil-ing water. Therefore not normally destroyed in cooking processes	Forms spores which can survive several hours in boiling water, therefore not normally destroyed in cooking processes

THE HUMAN DIGESTIVE SYSTEM

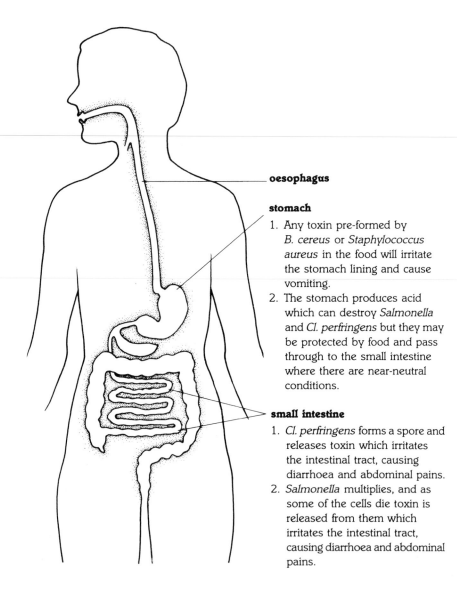

oesophagus

stomach

1. Any toxin pre-formed by
   B. cereus or *Staphylococcus
   aureus* in the food will irritate
   the stomach lining and cause
   vomiting.
2. The stomach produces acid
   which can destroy *Salmonella*
   and *Cl. perfringens* but they may
   be protected by food and pass
   through to the small intestine
   where there are near-neutral
   conditions.

small intestine

1. *Cl. perfringens* forms a spore and
   releases toxin which irritates
   the intestinal tract, causing
   diarrhoea and abdominal pains.
2. *Salmonella* multiplies, and as
   some of the cells die toxin is
   released from them which
   irritates the intestinal tract,
   causing diarrhoea and abdominal
   pains.

Chapter 10

Personal Hygiene and Kitchen Hygiene

There are two aspects to the prevention of food poisoning.

1. A food handler must as far as possible prevent bacteria from entering food by maintaining a high standard of personal hygiene and by being aware of all possible sources of contamination in the kitchen.

2. A food handler must discourage the multiplication of any bacteria which may be present so that the numbers never become sufficiently large to cause an outbreak of food poisoning. This can be done by cooking and storing foods correctly (see chapter 11).

HAND WASHING

Food poisoning bacteria carried on the hands and transferred into food during its preparation are one of the most common causes of food poisoning.

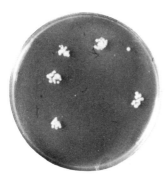

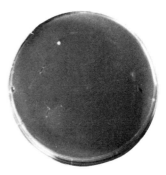

Before washing

After washing

Nutrient agar plates showing bacteria originating from unwashed and washed hands

In all catering establishments, by law, there must be sufficient wash basins in places where the food handlers can reach them quickly and easily from where they are working. Wash basins and nail brushes must also be provided near the toilets. Wash hand-basins should not be used for food washing and hands should not be washed in sinks used for the preparation of food or for washing-up.

Before commencing food preparation, hands and forearms should always be washed with hot water and soap and not just rinsed under the tap. A liquid soap dispenser is more hygienic than a soap tablet which is used by everybody. Some soaps are called bactericidal soaps because they contain a disinfectant which helps to reduce the number of bacteria on the hands.

Nails should always be kept short and should be scrubbed whenever the hands are washed because bacteria will collect under them. Nail varnish should not be worn when preparing foods as it easily chips and could fall into food.

Towels rapidly become contaminated with bacteria and an individual method of hand drying is essential. This can either be paper towels together with a foot operated disposal bin, a linen roller towel or a hot-air drier.

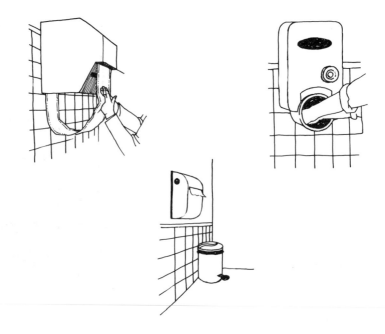

Hygienic methods of hand drying

After thorough drying, hand cream with added disinfectant should be used to keep the skin in good condition. Cracks and grooves in the skin surface or round the nails or knuckles usually harbour *Staphylococci* bacteria which are not easily removed when the hands are washed.

Hands must always be washed before handling food but even so unnecessary handling of food should be avoided. Where possible clean serving tongs should be used, especially for foods which are to be eaten without further cooking, e.g. cream cakes, cooked meats.

It is very important to wash the hands after:

Reason

1. Visiting the W.C.

Bacteria in the faeces can get through toilet paper on to the hands and so on to food.

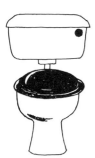

2. Blowing the nose.

Many people harbour *Staphylococci* bacteria in their noses. Some of these bacteria will be transferred to the hands when a handkerchief is handled. It is preferable to use disposable handkerchiefs which are destroyed after *one* use.

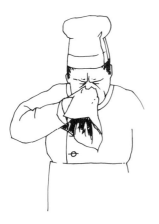

3. Handling raw meat, poultry or vegetables.

The transfer of bacteria from raw meat to cooked dishes (cross-contamination) is a frequent cause of food poisoning. Many raw meat samples have food poisoning bacteria (usually *Cl. perfringens* or *Salmonella*) on the surface. Soil usually contains spores of *Cl. perfringens.*

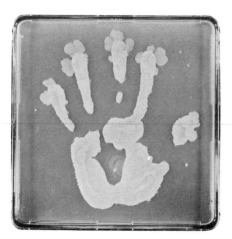

Nutrient agar plate showing presence of bacteria on the hand after handling raw meat

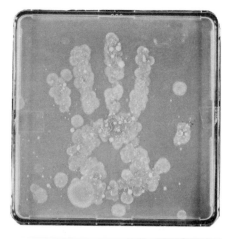

Nutrient agar plate showing presence of bacteria on the hand after washing vegetables coated with soil

4. Breaking eggs.

Salmonella is often present on eggshells.

5. After handling refuse or contaminated food.

A great number of all types of bacteria will be present in refuse and waste food.

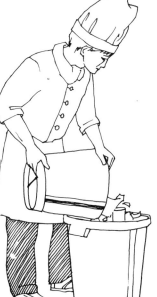

Under no circumstances should food handlers:

1. Smoke in the kitchen.

Reason

It is forbidden by law because bacteria can be transferred from the mouth and lips to the hands. Also, ash may drop into the food.

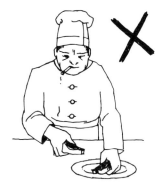

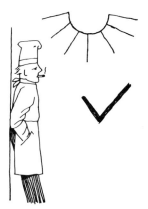

2. Sneeze or cough over food.   Droplets of moisture expelled during coughing and sneezing carry large numbers of *Staphylococci* bacteria to the food or working surfaces.

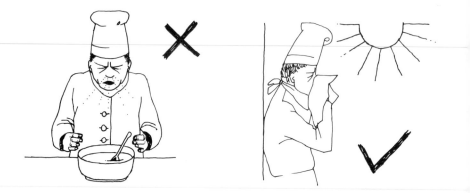

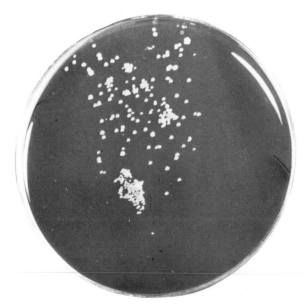

Nutrient agar plate showing bacterial growth produced by a sneeze

3. Comb their hair in the kitchen.

Staphylococci bacteria grow well on the scalp and will be transferred to the hands. Loose hairs and dandruff could fall on nearby food. Hair must be washed regularly and covered with a net or hat whilst working in the kitchen.

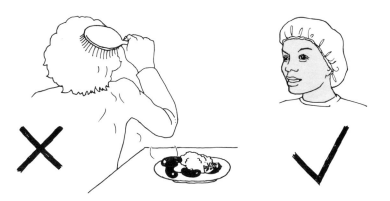

4. Dip their fingers into food to taste it, lick a spoon and return it to the food without washing it, or lick their fingers to separate sheets of wrapping paper.

Bacteria will be transferred from the mouth to the hands, spoon or paper and so to food.

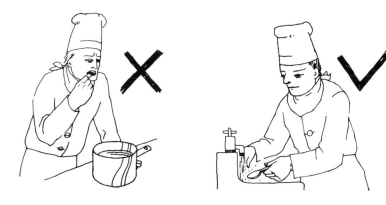

5. Wear any jewellery other than plain wedding rings whilst working in the kitchen.

The skin under jewellery tends to harbour a large number of bacteria especially if the jewellery is not removed in washing. There is always a risk that earrings, tie pins, cufflinks, dress rings, etc. could fall off and become mixed with the food.

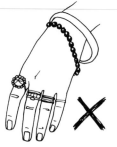

It is the duty of every food handler to:

1. Cover cuts and sores with a coloured waterproof dressing which must be changed regularly. Anyone with a septic cut or a boil, whitlow or stye should stop working with food until it is completely healed.

Reason

Any cut or sore is likely to be harbouring *Staphylococci* bacteria. If a coloured dressing accidentally falls off it will be seen before the food is used. If this does happen all the food in the same container must be discarded. It is not satisfactory merely to remove the dressing from the food. Septic cuts, boils, styes, and whitlows contain millions of *Staphylococci* bacteria.

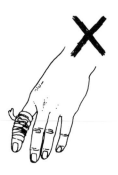

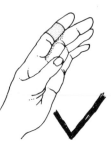

2. To report any illness, however mild, to the supervisor who will decide whether he is fit to work. This applies particularly to diarrhoea and vomiting, throat and skin infections.

Diarrhoea and vomiting are symptoms of food poisoning and even if the condition has cleared up, the employee may still be a convalescent carrier. *Staphylococci* bacteria are normally present in throat and skin infections.

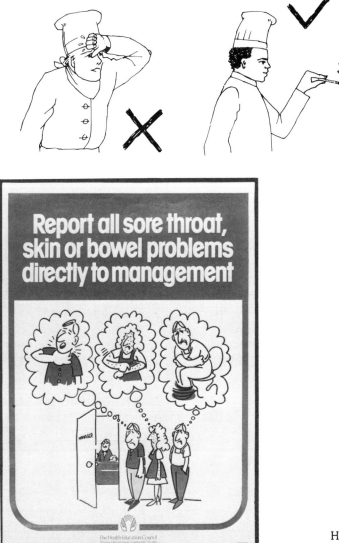

Health Education
Council poster

3. Wear clean overalls, aprons and headgear. Keep sleeves rolled up or securely fastened at the wrists so that cuffs cannot dip into food.

Outdoor clothing is frequently contaminated with *Staphylococci* particularly if it has been worn in congested areas such as on public transport. Clothing lockers should be situated outside the kitchen, making it possible to change into clean, protective clothing before handling food.

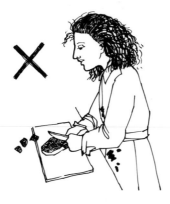

4. Use clean utensils for food preparation. Separate work surfaces and chopping boards should be set aside for the preparation of raw meat and must not be used for the preparation of foods which will be eaten without further cooking.

The transfer of bacteria from raw food to cooked food via kitchen utensils or work surfaces is frequently a cause of food poisoning.

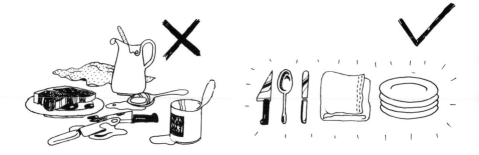

5. Pick up knives and forks by their handles, glasses by the stems and plates by the edges.

Bacteria on the hands can be passed to cutlery and crockery and from these articles back to food.

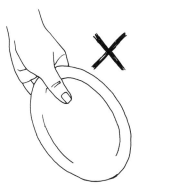 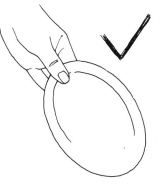

6. Discard any chipped plates, glasses and damaged utensils.

Even an efficient washing-up process may fail to remove bacteria from cracks.

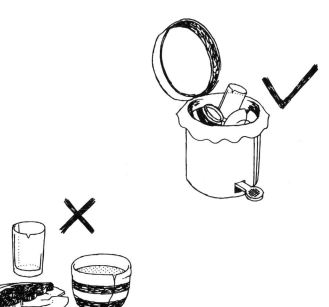

7. Cover food on display.

Flies will be attracted to uncovered food and bacteria in dust particles will settle on the food if it is left uncovered.

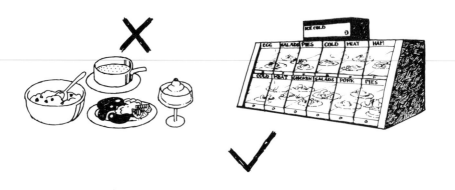

8. Keep pets out of the kitchen.

All animals carry bacteria on their feet and in their fur and these can easily spread into food if the animals are allowed to wander freely in the kitchen.

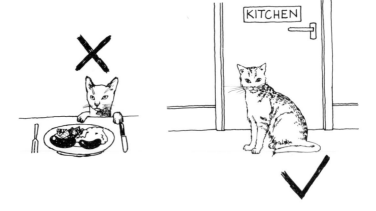

9. Keep pet food away from human food, using separate utensils for its preparation.

Pet food (except canned pet food) is usually heavily contaminated with bacteria.

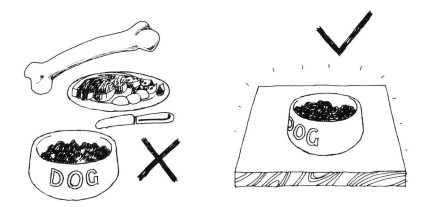

SUMMARY

Maintaining a high standard of personal cleanliness and reporting all illnesses will reduce the risk of causing food poisoning.

Chapter 11

The Control of Bacterial Growth

If the precautions listed in Chapter 10 are observed during food preparation there should be very few harmful bacteria added to the food and certainly not a sufficiently large number to cause food poisoning. However, the following precautions should be taken so that if some pathogenic bacteria were originally present in the food or have inadvertently entered during preparation, they will be prevented from multiplying.

1. Thaw all frozen meat completely before cooking

It is essential that all frozen meats (particularly poultry) should be thawed completely before commencing cooking. If ice is present in the centre of meat it will take far longer for the internal temperature to reach that of the external temperature than in completely defrosted meat. *Salmonella* food poisoning has frequently been caused because chickens have not been thoroughly defrosted. Although they have been cooked for the recommended time, a great deal of heat is used to melt the remaining ice and the temperature reached in the centre of the bird is not sufficiently high to kill *Salmonella* but is an optimum temperature for its multiplication.

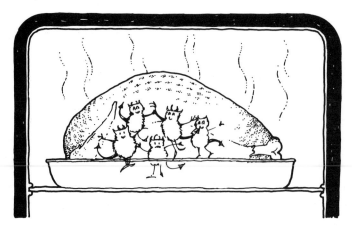

2. Cook food thoroughly

Food is a poor conductor of heat and it takes a long time before the temperature in the centre reaches the same temperature as at the surface. For this reason it is safer to reduce the size of rolled joints and minced meats to a maximum of 6 lb before cooking them.

Meat and meat products containing raw meat should never be partly cooked one day and the cooking process finished the next day. If the food is only partly cooked it is likely that bacteria will still be alive, and even if it is stored in a refrigerator there will be time for bacteria to multiply during the cooling down process and the second heating process. Just as the centre of joints of meat and meat products only slowly reaches the external temperature when heated up, the temperature at the centre of a hot product drops much more slowly than the temperature at the surface.

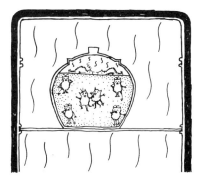

If food has been deep frozen and thawed it must not be refrozen for the same reason. Bacteria are not often killed by deep freeze temperatures and when the food is thawed they will have a chance to multiply. If the food is then refrozen, a greatly increased number of bacteria will be present, all capable of multiplying next time it is thawed.

3. Cool food quickly and keep it cold until it is ready to be served or reheated

All foods should be cooled as quickly as possible so that harmful bacteria will have only a short time at a temperature at which they can multiply. Cooked food should not be taken straight from the oven and put into the refrigerator, however, as this will increase the temperature of the refrigerator to a dangerously high level, and food poisoning bacteria may be able to multiply in other foods being stored there.

Place hot cooked foods in a cold room for approximately one hour and then put them in the refrigerator. To speed up the cooling process, large volumes of meat can be divided and cooled in smaller containers.

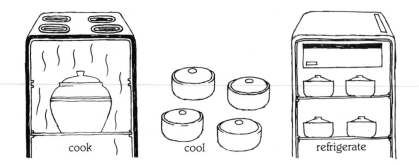

cook   cool   refrigerate

4. Never keep food warm

Keep food either very hot or very cold. Do not keep it in a warm atmosphere, e.g. a service counter, as this will allow the rapid multiplication of bacteria. If food is to be served hot it should be served as soon as possible after cooking and provided the temperature is kept above 63 °C (145 °F) there is little danger of bacteria multiplying.

If food is to be served cold, it should be stored in a refrigerator until just before it is served.

These rules are particularly important if the food concerned is susceptible to bacterial growth e.g. meats and meat products, gravies, milk and cream products.

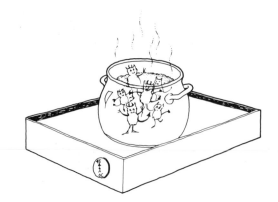

5. Never reheat food more than once

Reheating food is always a hazard because cooked food may still contain spores of *Cl. perfringens* or *B. cereus* or it may have been contaminated with any type of bacteria after cooking. When the food is cooled the spores will germinate and start to multiply along with any other bacteria present. When the food is warmed up, the temperatures used are not normally high enough to destroy toxins or to kill spore-forming bacteria.

If reheating is absolutely necessary, the food should be covered and cooled very rapidly after cooking and stored in a refrigerator until it is ready to be reheated. It should then be reheated rapidly and thoroughly. Hot gravy or sauce should never be added to cold food in order to heat it up, since the combined temperature will probably be optimum for bacterial growth.

Under no circumstances should meat products or rice be reheated more than once because each time a food is reheated there are two opportunities for bacteria to multiply, once during the heating up process and once during the cooling down process. In schools and hospitals the usual policy is not to reheat foods at all, since children and sick people are particularly susceptible to food poisoning.

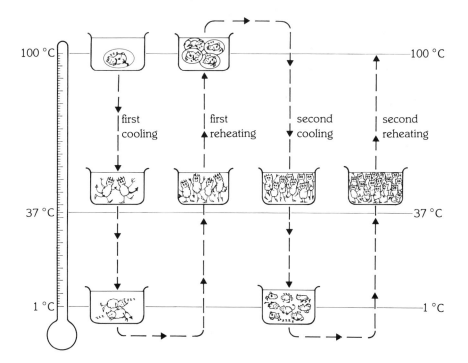

Factors contributing to 1479 outbreaks of food poisoning in England and Wales 1970-1982

| Contributing factor | Number of outbreaks in which factor recorded | | | | | |
	Salmonella	*Cl. perfringens*	*S. aureus*	*B. cereus*	*Other*	Total (%)
Preparation too far in advance	240	464	80	54	6	844 (25)
Storage at ambient temperature	172	276	75	39	4	566 (17)
Inadequate cooling	125	313	12	17	1	468 (14)
Inadequate reheating	76	275	5	33	2	391 (12)
Contaminated processed food	100	19	27	4	86	236 (7)
Undercooking	139	74	2	1	7	223 (7)
Contaminated canned food	2	4	42	1	55	104 (3)
Inadequate thawing	61	34	—	—	—	95 (3)
Cross-contamination	84	8	2	—	—	94 (3)
Raw food consumed	84	—	1	—	8	93 (3)
Improper warm holding	15	52	—	8	2	77 (2)
Infected food handlers	13	—	50	—	2	65 (2)
Use of left overs	25	25	11	1	—	62 (2)
Extra large quantities prepared	29	17	2	—	—	48 (1)
Total	1165	1561	309	158	173	3366

Source: PHLS Communicable Disease Surveillance Centre
Extracted from Diane Roberts 'Factors contributing to outbreaks of food poisoning in England and Wales 1970-1979', The Journal of Hygiene, volume 89, 1982, pp. 491-8. (updated) (Totals do not correlate because several factors may contribute to one outbreak.)

SUMMARY

1. All frozen meat should be thoroughly thawed before cooking.

2. Food must be kept either very hot or very cold before it is served and never left in a warm temperature for any length of time.

3. The practice of reheating food should be avoided wherever possible. Meat products and rice must never be reheated more than once.

Chapter 12

Temperature Control of Food

The previous chapter explained the importance of keeping food either very hot (above 63 °C (145 °F)) or very cold (below 10 °C (50 °F)). Most kitchens have refrigerators, freezers and sometimes cool rooms for low temperature storage and some means of keeping food very hot when it is soon to be served. In addition, microwave ovens are frequently used to reheat foods quickly. The successful use of various combinations of this equipment will ensure that food spends very little time at a temperature at which bacteria will multiply.

REFRIGERATORS

Operating temperature

A refrigerator should operate at a temperature between 1 °C and 4 °C (34 °F and 40 °F). Pathogenic bacteria will not multiply at this temperature but they will not be killed. During refrigerated storage, food poisoning bacteria remain dormant but as soon as the food is removed from the refrigerator and put in a warm room they will start to multiply rapidly. Many food spoilage bacteria are able to multiply in the refrigerator but at a much slower rate than at room temperature.

To maintain the correct temperature it is important to:

1. Keep the door shut whenever possible.

2. Cool hot foods before putting them in the refrigerator. Hot foods would cause a considerable increase in the temperature and also condensation which may lead to cross-contamination.

3. Defrost regularly. Defrosting is the removal of excess ice which forms around the refrigerating coils and reduces their efficiency.

The temperature of the refrigerator should not be allowed to drop below 1 °C because ice crystals would form in the food causing loss of texture and quality.

Position of foods

The position of foods in a refrigerator should be carefully planned so that cross-contamination will not occur. Raw meat, poultry, vegetables and fish should be stored separately from prepared food which will not be cooked again. If there is more than one refrigerator in the kitchen, different ones can be used for raw and cooked foods. If there is only one, raw foods should be stored at the bottom of the refrigerator and cooked foods at the top so that contaminated blood or food particles cannot drop from the raw foods to the cooked foods. Strong-smelling foods such as fish should be put in an airtight container and placed as far away as possible from foods which readily absorb smells, such as butter.

Covering of foods in the refrigerator prevents drying out, cross-contamination and the absorption of odours. Cling film is useful for this purpose but should not be placed over the food until it has cooled. The condensation which collects when cling film is placed over warm food speeds up spoilage of that food.

A refrigerator functions by circulating cold air round the food so it is essential that it is not so tightly packed that the circulation of air is restricted.

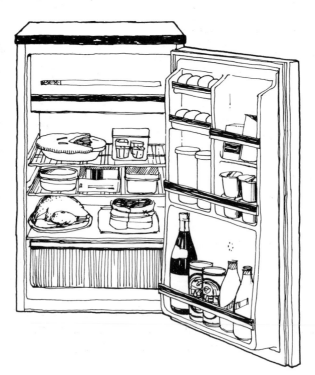

There have been many recent developments in refrigeration units for use in large catering establishments. The basic unit is the 'reach-in' cabinet which is available in many sizes. Any combination of removable internal fittings such as shelves or deep containers can be chosen depending on storage requirements. All these are removable to facilitate cleaning. Stainless steel doors are usually fitted to withstand tough treatment in busy kitchens. The illustration below shows a modern service cabinet.

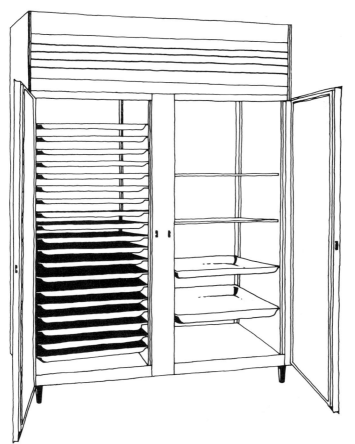

For even larger quantities, 'roll-in' refrigerators are available which will accommodate trolleys of food. Some have a door at the preparations end and a door at the opposite end which opens in the serving area.

Other refrigeration units include mobile refrigerators for food which is to be served a distance from the preparation area and refrigerators with glass doors which can be used for displaying food such as cream cakes and wine.

CHILLERS

A refrigerator should not be used to cool hot food, and in a catering establishment where large volumes of food such as roast meats and poultry must be cooled quickly before refrigerating a blast chiller is almost essential. The temperature of the food is reduced quickly due to the circulation of a continuous current of cold air.

FREEZERS

Operating temperature

The length of time which food can be safely stored in a freezer depends on the temperature of the freezer. A star marking system has been devised which indicates the temperature of the freezer and consequently the time for which food may be stored.

The star marking system for frozen food compartments

	temperature of freezer	food storage time
✻	−6 °C (21 °F)	1 week
✻✻	−12 °C (10 °F)	1 month
✻✻✻	−18 °C (0 °F)	3 months
✱ ✻✻✻	−18 °C (0 °F) to −25 °C (−15 °C)	3 months or longer; capable of freezing fresh food

Most domestic freezers operate at −18 °C and are capable of freezing fresh food without affecting the temperature of the frozen food already in the cabinet. Some bacteria will be killed during storage at this temperature but many can remain dormant for long periods of time. Spores and toxins are not affected by deep freezing. When food is taken out of the deep freeze and thawed, the surviving bacteria start to grow and multiply again. Food that has been frozen tends to allow more rapid bacterial growth than the equivalent fresh food and therefore deteriorates rather more quickly.

Refreezing

Food should not be refrozen once it has thawed unless it is cooked in between. There are two reasons for this:

1. If the thawed food is kept at a temperature above 10 °C for some time, any pathogenic bacteria present will have a chance to multiply.

2. The texture of the food will suffer. Large ice crystals tend to form when food is frozen relatively slowly in domestic freezers. The loss of texture which this causes is more noticeable in food which has been thawed and refrozen.

Freezer breakdown

If there is a power cut or the freezer breaks down, the door or lid should be kept closed and covered with blankets to minimize the temperature increase. If the food is still partially frozen when the power is restored or the freezer is mended, it may be safe to refreeze the food. If in doubt, an environmental health officer will give advice on this matter. If the food has completely thawed out, one of the following options must be chosen:

1. Use the food immediately.

2. Store the food in a refrigerator but for no longer than 2 days.

3. Cook the food thoroughly, cool rapidly and store in a refrigerator for no longer than 3 days.

4. Destroy the food.

MICROWAVE OVENS

Cooking and reheating of foods in microwave ovens is now common practice in many catering establishments. Generally speaking, using a microwave oven is a safe way of cooking and reheating foods and eliminates many of the problems of conventional reheating, but it is important that food is stored correctly beforehand. Heating in a microwave oven will destroy most vegetative bacteria but will not destroy toxins formed by them, or spores. It is therefore not satisfactory to reheat meat products or rice more than once.

It can be useful to make a table which gives the correct setting and the time required for adequate heating of the foods most frequently handled. The time required will depend on the density of the food and the quantity present in the oven.

Most microwave ovens have a defrost cycle for thawing frozen food. If not, to ensure even thawing, defrosting must be achieved by a microwave cook followed by a resting phase.

This type of table is useful in a catering establishment where a microwave oven is used.

Food	Setting	Time
Trout (6 oz)	Defrost	2½ min
Chicken joint (8 oz)	Defrost	3 min
Plated meal (16 oz)	Defrost	5½ min
Frozen sandwich	Defrost	1½ min
Meat pie (5 oz)	Heating	25 sec
Meat pie (5 oz) × 5	Heating	1¼ min
Plated meal (16 oz)	Heating	1½ min
Apple pie — 8 portions	Heating	3½ min
Pizza (8 in)	Heating	40 sec
Pizza (8 in) × 4	Heating	60 sec
Chicken (3 lb 6 oz)	Cooking	16 min
Trout (6 oz)	Cooking	1 min
Frozen peas (2 lb)	Cooking	4½ min

HOLDING UNITS

Many kitchens have a hot cupboard and/or a *bain-marie* for keeping food warm for short periods of time just before it is served. A hot cupboard is heated by gas or electricity and a *bain-marie* is a heated well filled with hot water. Both systems should be hot enough to ensure that the temperature at the centre of the food is kept above 63 °C (145 °F). They must never be used for heating up cold foods as the process would be too slow using either piece of equipment.

COOK-CHILL AND COOK-FREEZE SYSTEMS

These methods of food preparation are becoming increasingly common and are widely used where centralised catering is practised.

The food usually has to be transported a long distance from the kitchens where it is prepared, e.g. aeroplane meals, school meals, hospital meals. In any of these situations it would be unsatisfactory to cook the food and keep it warm until it is required.

In cook-chill and cook-freeze systems the food is prepared in the central preparation unit: it is cooked thoroughly and then divided into individual portions observing strict hygiene standards. All containers are marked with the date (to ensure effective stock rotation) and also with the contents, reheating time and any other instructions.

Cook-chill The food is chilled to between 1 °C and 3 °C (33–37 °F) within two hours of cooking and must be kept in a refrigerator at this temperature until it is required for distribution. It should be reheated to 70 °C within two hours of arrival at the point of consumption. All meals must be eaten within five days including the day of preparation.

There is no danger of cook-chill foods causing food poisoning if these conditions are met. Recently a bacterium called *Listeria monocytogenes* which does not cause food poisoning but can cause meningitis has been found in a few samples of cook-chill foods. It is capable of growing at refrigeration temperatures but will be destroyed provided the food is reheated thoroughly.

Cook-freeze The food is blast-frozen (a very rapid method of freezing) to a temperature of − 18 °C (0 °F) and kept at this temperature until required. It must be reheated to 70 °C or above.

Whichever system is used, any reheated food which is not consumed must be discarded.

It is important to bear in mind that any departure from these guidelines could result in an outbreak of food poisoning involving a large number of people. Further details can be obtained from the DHSS code of practice *Guidelines on pre-cooked chilled foods.*

SUMMARY

1. The temperature of a refrigerator must be maintained between 1 °C and 4 °C (34 °F and 40 °F).
2. Frozen food should not be refrozen once it has thawed.
3. Microwave ovens are very useful for quick reheating of food.
4. Holding units must not be used for heating up cold foods.
5. The cook-chill and cook-freeze methods of food preparation are useful when food has to be cooked some distance from where it is to be served.

Chapter 13

Foods Most Likely to Cause Food Poisoning

Some foods favour the growth of food poisoning bacteria; others do not.

When food poisoning is confirmed it is not always easy to identify the food which has caused the outbreak as there are frequently no samples of the suspected foods left. However, certain foods are regarded as being 'high-risk' and, if eaten just before the illness, will be suspected as the cause. In some of the investigated outbreaks sufficient evidence is available to implicate one particular food.

Foods implicated in 194 outbreaks of food poisoning in 1983

Food	Salmonella	Clostridium perfringens	Staphylococcus aureus	Bacillus cereus	Total
Chicken	36	8	5	2	51
Turkey	9	8	0	0	17
Poultry (not specified)	0	1	0	0	1
Beef	7	16	0	1	24
Pork/ham	4	5	2	0	11
Lamb	1	3	0	0	4
Other meats and pies	18	12	1	1	32
Gravy/sauces	0	1	0	0	1
Rice	0	0	0	9	9
Milk	13	0	0	0	13
Cheese	0	0	1	0	1
Egg	1	0	1	0	2
Fish	1	0	2	0	3
Other/ mixed foods	9	10	2	4	25
Totals	99	64	14	17	194

Source: PHLS Communicable Disease Surveillance Centre
Extracted from 'Food poisoning and Salmonella surveillance in England and Wales 1983', British Medical Journal, volume 291, pp. 394-6.

HIGH-RISK FOODS

Foods which encourage the growth of bacteria are usually high in protein and moisture. Examples are meat, poultry, eggs, milk and any foods where these are ingredients. Special precautions must be taken when preparing high-risk foods to ensure that:

1. They are not contaminated during preparation especially if they will be eaten uncooked or after only gently heating.

2. They are not left in a warm temperature for any longer than is absolutely necessary for their preparation so that there will be little time for any bacteria present to multiply. They should be served hot (above 63 °C (145 °F)) or cold (straight from the refrigerator).

MEAT AND MEAT PRODUCTS

Every year the majority of food poisoning outbreaks are caused by meat and meat products.

Freshly roasted meat

Freshly roasted or grilled meat, served hot immediately after cooking, is rarely a cause of food poisoning. Even a rare steak is safe because bacteria are not present in the centre of the meat, only on the surface.

Chickens

It is estimated that 80% of raw chickens carry *Salmonella*. However, freshly roasted chickens or other poultry will cause food poisoning only if they have been cooked for less than the recommended time or if they were not completely defrosted before cooking.

Rolled joints

Rolled joints are more frequently a cause of food poisoning because surface meat which may be contaminated will be at the centre of the joint after rolling and also considerable handling by the chef is necessary. It is therefore essential that rolled joints should be small enough to allow sufficient heat to kill bacteria to penetrate to the centre during cooking.

Cold meats

Cold meats are frequently a cause of food poisoning usually because they have been contaminated after cooking and kept in a warm environment for several hours before serving.

Stews and casseroles

If served hot immediately after cooking, stews and casseroles will not cause food poisoning. If they are kept warm for several hours or cooled slowly and reheated the next day, there is far more chance that they will cause food poisoning because any spores of *Cl. perfringens* which survived the first cooking process will have had time to germinate and multiply.

Minced meat

When meat is minced, any pathogenic bacteria which were present on the surface are distributed throughout the mass of the meat. Only sufficient meat to provide a day's supply should be minced at any one time.

Pies, pasties, rissoles, sausages and other 'made-up' meat dishes

'Made-up' meat dishes are frequently a cause of food poisoning because bacteria may be present throughout the food. Care must be taken to cook sufficiently to kill any bacteria in the centre.

Stocks

Stocks will not cause food poisoning if they are served hot because they have usually been boiling for several hours. If they have been kept warm and then reheated rapidly before serving, they are a likely cause of food poisoning. For the same reason it is important to keep gravies, soups and sauces very hot (above 63 °C (145 °F)) until just before they are served.

Gelatin

Powdered gelatin frequently contains dormant food poisoning bacteria. When it is melted in water for use in meat pies or as a glaze it becomes an ideal food for bacterial growth and must therefore be kept at a temperature above 63 °C (145 °F) until it is used.

FISH

Freshly cooked fish is rarely a cause of food poisoning because food poisoning bacteria are not usually present in the intestines of cold-blooded animals. Shellfish have been known to cause food poisoning because they have been gathered from polluted waters but there are now laws governing the gathering and cleansing of them. Fish dishes such as fish cakes or fish pie may be contaminated during preparation and should therefore always be stored correctly and reheated thoroughly.

DAIRY PRODUCTS

Milk

Most milk for sale in this country has been pasteurised which means that it is free of pathogenic bacteria. However, milk is an ideal food for bacterial growth and could cause food poisoning if contaminated after pasteurisation. Any dishes where milk is an ingredient, such as custards, trifles, milk puddings and sauces, must be served hot or refrigerated until served. Raw (unpasteurised) milk has caused several outbreaks of food poisoning.

Cream

Cream for sale in this country has been pasteurised. Cream, like milk, is an ideal food for bacterial growth if it is contaminated after pasteurisation. All cream cakes, trifles etc. should be kept cold until just before they are served. The same precautions must be taken with imitation cream.

Evaporated milk

Evaporated milk is safe when the can is first opened but supports the growth of bacteria and if not used straight away should be stored in the refrigerator.

Condensed milk

The high sugar content of condensed milk makes it unsuitable for bacterial growth.

Dried milk

Dried milk powder contains many dormant bacteria. Once reconstituted it must be treated as fresh milk and stored in the refrigerator.

Ice cream

Ice cream purchased from a reputable supplier can be regarded as safe. Ice cream should not be thawed and then refrozen.

Cheese

In Britain, cheese is normally made from pasteurised milk and is therefore rarely a cause of food poisoning. Hard cheeses do not contain sufficient moisture for bacterial growth, but low-fat cheeses do and if contaminated after manufacture could be a cause of food poisoning.

EGGS

Raw egg is ideal for bacterial growth. A small proportion of hen eggs carry *Salmonella* inside the shell. It is therefore preferable to cook eggs thoroughly especially if they are to be eaten by an elderly, very young or sick person since these people would be more seriously affected by food poisoning.

Duck eggs are more frequently contaminated with *Salmonella* inside the shell and should always be thoroughly cooked.

Egg shells are often contaminated so care must be taken to prevent transfer of bacteria from the shell to the raw egg or any other food in the kitchen.

RICE

Rice is often contaminated with *B. cereus* which forms spores capable of surviving the cooking process. If rice is not eaten immediately after cooking it must be stored in the refrigerator.

LOW-RISK FOODS

Certain foods do not normally cause food poisoning because they do not provide bacteria with the nutrients they require for growth and multiplication. Foods with a high concentration of sugar, salt, acid or fat or dry foods will not support the growth of food poisoning bacteria.

Jams, syrup, honey, salted meat, anchovies

These foods are unlikely to cause food poisoning because the sugar/salt concentration is too high. The sugar and salt present in the food dissolve in the water to form a concentrated solution leaving insufficient moisture for bacterial growth.

Fatty foods

Very few types of bacteria can multiply in the presence of high concentrations of fat and those which can are not the ones that cause food poisoning.

Acid foods

Food poisoning bacteria will not grow in very acid foods such as pickles and citrus fruits.

Dry foods

Dry foods will not support the growth of food poisoning bacteria but may contain them. If water is added at a later stage in preparation the bacteria will be able to multiply again so the food must then be treated as fresh food and stored in a refrigerator.

Canned foods

In Britain, food is canned and sterilised under strict control and any manufactured canned food can be regarded as safe unless the can is damaged. If it is punctured, has a faulty seam or swollen ends (caused by gas produced inside the can) the manufacturer should be notified and the can and contents either returned or thrown away. Canned ham is often pasteurised only, since sterilisation affects the quality of the ham; it must therefore be stored in a refrigerator. After canned food has been opened it should be handled and stored as fresh food.

SUMMARY

1. Moist, high protein foods will usually support the growth of food poisoning bacteria.

2. Foods with a high concentration of sugar, salt, acid or fat or dry foods will not support the growth of food poisoning bacteria.

Chapter 14

How Common is Food Poisoning?

The number of reported cases of food poisoning is showing an increase in most years despite higher standards of hygiene and increased awareness of the causes of food poisoning. Notified food poisoning cases in England and Wales increased from 9195 in 1977 to 15 168 in 1983. It is estimated that there are at least ten times as many cases which are not reported and are therefore not included in these figures.

Laboratory reports (all cases) for England and Wales: 1977–83

Organism	1977	1978	1979	1980	1981	1982	1983
Salmonella	6501	9086	9912	9540	9532	11 099	13 250
Cl. perfringens	2576	1024	1607	1056	918	1455	1624
S. aureus	81	301	328	189	143	89	160
B. cereus	37	143	22	64	72	41	134
Totals	9195	10 572	11 869	10 849	10 665	12 684	15 168

Source: PHLS Communicable Disease Surveillance Centre

There are a number of reasons for this increase:

1. Intensive rearing of farm animals such as chickens and pigs. The concentrated feeds which are given to them are frequently contaminated with *Salmonella*, and because the animals are so crowded, bacteria can easily spread from one to another. The meat we buy is therefore often contaminated with pathogenic bacteria.

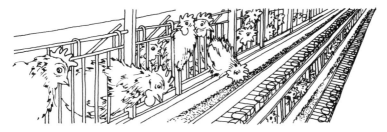

2. The practice of eating out is becoming far more popular and the majority of the working population is eating at least one meal a day in a restaurant, pub or canteen. If a mistake is made in food preparation in one of these catering establishments a large number of people will be affected, whereas a similar incident in the home will affect only a small number of people.

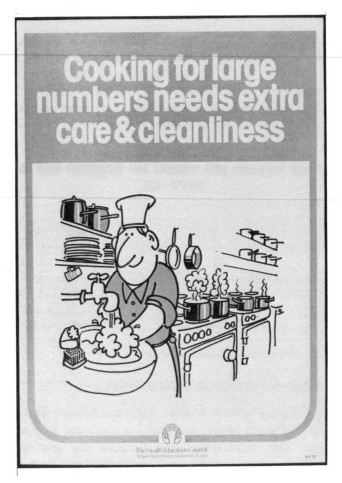

Health Education Council poster

3. Restaurants, canteens etc. produce a much more varied range of dishes than used to be the case. With this degree of choice, instead of food being served hot immediately after it is cooked, there is tendency to keep foods warm until a customer requests a particular dish. The increasing use of microwave ovens will hopefully reduce cases of food poisoning caused by keeping food warm.

```
┌─────────────────────────────────────────┐
│  ∿∿∿∿∿∿  MENU  ∿∿∿∿∿∿                     │
│                                          │
│  Chili con carne              1·70       │
│                                          │
│  Hungarian goulash            1·65       │
│                                          │
│  Moussaka                     1·90       │
│                                          │
│  Sweet and sour pork          2·00       │
│                                          │
│  Lasagne                      1·80       │
│                                          │
│  Chicken and prawn pilaff     2·10       │
│                                          │
│  Beef and mushroom pie        1·75       │
│                                          │
│  Spaghetti bolognese          1·75       │
│            ───────────//──────           │
│                                          │
│  Black Forest gâteau            75       │
│                                          │
│  Sherry trifle                  75       │
│                                          │
│  Chocolate mousse               70       │
└─────────────────────────────────────────┘
```

4. There has been a rapid growth in the number of shops selling take-away meals. The food is frequently cooked in advance and then reheated on purchase. If it is not cooled quickly and stored in a refrigerator between cooking and reheating there will be plenty of opportunity for bacterial growth.

TAKE-AWAY MENU

Chicken and chips	1.30	Lamb curry and rice	1.75
Steak pie and chips	90	Beef curry and rice	1.85
Cheeseburger	1.20	Special fried rice	1.20
Pizza	1.35	Sweet and sour pork	2.20
Barbecued spare ribs	1.95	Sweet and sour chicken	2.15
Jacket potato		Doner kebab	1.30
– with chicken	1.00	Shish kebab	1.40
– with prawns	1.20		

SERVED WITHIN 5 MINUTES OF ORDERING

5. Large-scale factory production of foods has led to an increase in food poisoning. Although factory processes are normally very carefully controlled, a slight error at some stage in production could lead to thousands of contaminated prepacked foods which may be distributed throughout the country.

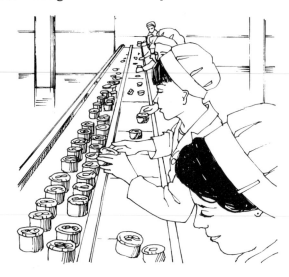

6. Many housewives now work full-time, hence shopping is probably done weekly rather than daily, resulting in a greater chance of bacterial growth in the food after purchase unless it is stored correctly. Meals are sometimes cooked ahead of requirements and reheated when needed which increases the chance for bacterial growth.

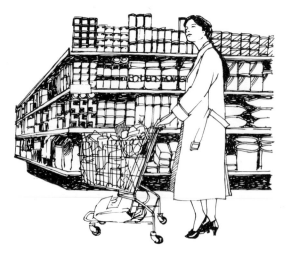

7. The majority of outbreaks of food poisoning occur during the summer months. The hot summer of 1983 caused an increase in the number of outbreaks. In the summer, there is an increased tendency to pack foods, e.g. for picnics and for journeys to holiday resorts. These are often kept at warm temperatures for several hours before they are eaten. Insulated bags and ice boxes should be used to keep food cool if it will not be eaten for several hours after removal from the refrigerator. Flies present a hygiene problem in the summer months.

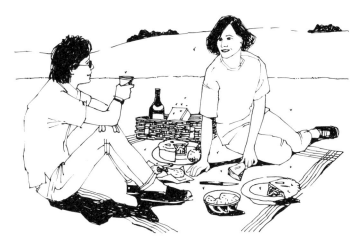

8. Untrained staff are often employed during the summer months to cope with the increased demand for restaurant meals. All staff should be taught the basic principles of food hygiene and should be carefully supervised in their first few weeks' work.

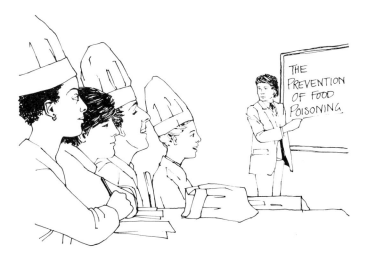

SUMMARY

1. The number of cases of food poisoning is increasing in most years due to:
    (a) Intensive rearing of farm animals.
    (b) An increased tendency to eat out.
    (c) A much more varied menu.
    (d) An increasing number of shops selling take-away meals.
    (e) Large scale factory production of food.
    (f) An increased tendency to shop and cook several days in advance of eating.

2. The majority of outbreaks of food poisoning occur in the summer months.

3. It is very important for all food handlers to be trained in food hygiene.

Chapter 15

Washing-up

The aim of washing-up is to remove visible food waste and to destroy the bacteria which will be present on dirty kitchen equipment. It is very important that all utensils, crockery, containers, etc. used for food should be thoroughly cleaned each time they are used. Many food poisoning outbreaks have occurred due to the use of kitchen equipment which is not clean. Hot water and chemicals are used for washing-up. The chemicals, known as detergents and disinfectants, perform different functions.

Detergents are chemicals which act with water to make things clean by allowing the whole surface, even if it is greasy, to become wet. If water alone is used, it tends to form droplets on a greasy surface.

THIS IS HOW DETERGENTS WORK

Stage I

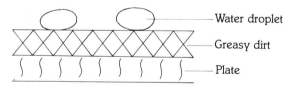

Water does not spread evenly on greasy plates and tends to form small droplets

Stage II

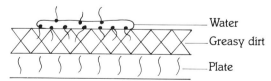

The water now spreads on the grease;
The detergent molecules 'fasten' the water and grease together;
Rubbing with a cloth or sponge removes grease and dirt together from the plate.

Stage III

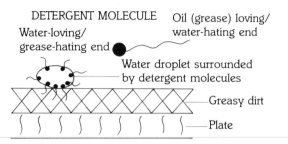

Detergent is added to the water;
The detergent molecules surround the water droplets;
The head of the molecule (water-loving end) enters the water;
The tail (water-hating end) is attracted to the grease.

Stage IV

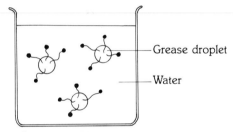

The grease now rolls up into drops surrounded by detergent molecules and is suspended in the water. When the water goes down the drain the grease goes with it.

Soap is an example of a simple detergent but it is not normally used for washing-up. Instead synthetic detergents (washing-up liquids) are used as they wet surfaces more effectively and do not form a scum with hard water.

A detergent does not kill bacteria but reduces the number present on an article by removing the dirt and grease which are harbouring the bacteria.

Disinfectants are chemicals which will kill the majority of bacteria present on surfaces and equipment, though not necessarily all of them. Spores will survive disinfection. However, disinfection of articles after washing with a detergent is sufficient to prevent food poisoning occurring.

Disinfection can also be achieved by the use of hot water. This has many advantages and should be used wherever possible.

Hypochlorites are chemicals which are often used as disinfectants for articles to be used for food preparation and storage. If they are used at the correct concentration they leave no taste or smell. The hotter the water, the more effective the disinfectant.

Sanitisers are chemicals which combine both a detergent and disinfectant. Chemical disinfectants are partially inactivated by dirt and food residues, so sanitisers are not as effective for dirty equipment and surfaces as a detergent wash followed by disinfection.

Sterilants are chemicals which will kill all bacteria and spores present on surfaces and equipment. Steam can be used for this purpose.

Antiseptics are chemicals which will kill or check the growth of bacteria present on or in the human body, e.g. Savlon, TCP.

Deodorants are chemicals which mask or hide odour but do not kill bacteria, e.g. fresh air sprays.

WASHING-UP PROCEDURE

Washing-up should not take place in a food preparation area because of the danger of dirty plates contaminating work surfaces which are to be used for the preparation of food. If a kitchen serves a canteen or restaurant, the washing-up area should be next to the restaurant so that dirty crockery and utensils need not be brought into the kitchen at all. Washing up can be done either by hand, in which case at least two sinks are necessary, or by a dish-washing machine. Whichever method is used, the process is similar and comprises three stages.

1. *Preparation*   Crockery should be scraped clean and if possible all crockery and utensils should be given a pre-rinse in warm water so that the washing water at the next stage will stay cleaner.

2. *Main wash*   At this stage a detergent is added to the water to help remove food remains and grease.

    The temperature of the water should be between 50 °C and 60 °C (122 °F and 140 °F). This is too hot for bare hands so rubber gloves will be needed. It should not exceed 63 °C (145 °F) because certain protein residues such as traces of egg become baked on to plates and cutlery if very hot water is used. Wiping with a clean dishcloth in this combination of hot water and detergent will remove grease and food residues but it will not make the equipment completely free from bacteria. It is best to use disposable dishcloths, but if more substantial ones are preferred they should be washed and dried daily.

The washing-up water must be changed frequently and more detergent added so it will always be both clean and at the correct temperature.

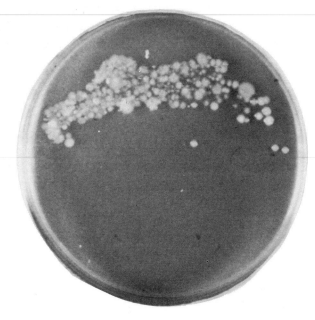

Nutrient agar plate showing bacteria present
in one drop of liquid from a dirty dishcloth

3. *Rinsing stage*   The articles are transferred from the sink which contains water and detergent into a sink containing very hot water at a temperature of about 80 °C (176 °F). They are left immersed in the water for 2 minutes. The purpose of this stage is:

   (a) to rinse off any traces of detergent. Detergents left on plates could affect the flavour of food put on them and may possibly cause harmful effects if they are ingested over a long period of time;

   (b) to kill any remaining bacteria;

   (c) to heat the articles to a sufficiently high temperature to allow them to air dry.

This rinsing process will only be performed effectively if the temperature is maintained at 80 °C (176 °F). If this is not possible, a chemical disinfectant should be added to the rinsing water to destroy the bacteria which are still present after the detergent wash.

4. *Drying* It is generally considered best to allow crockery and utensils to drain dry in racks. They will dry fairly quickly if the temperature of the rinse water is maintained at 80 °C (176 °F). If tea towels are used, a clean one must be used for each washing-up session because a moist dirty tea towel in a warm kitchen is an ideal place for bacteria to grow. Clean, dry crockery and utensils should be stored under cover so that they will not be re-contaminated.

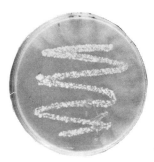

Nutrient agar plates showing bacteria present on a chopping board after preparing raw meat

Without washing

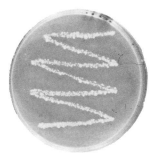

After wiping with a dishcloth

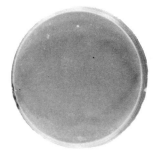

After correct washing-up

Dish-washing machines

There are many different types of dish-washing machines all of which vary slightly in their operation. It is therefore important to follow the manufacturer's instructions. The principle is the same as for the hand-washing method. Dirty crockery and utensils are stacked into the machine, pre-rinsed, washed in water at 60 °C (140 °F) and a detergent, and then rinsed at a temperature between 80 °C and 88 °C (176–190 °F). They should be allowed to air-dry under cover.

It is essential that regular checks are made to ensure that the dish-washing machine is working correctly. Most machines have dials on the outside so that the operator can check that the temperatures of the water are correct and that the articles are exposed to the very hot rinsing water for the correct length of time.

Glassware

Glassware should be washed by a two-stage method with detergent and water at 50–60 °C (122–140 °F) in the first sink and water at 80 °C (176 °F) in the second sink. If the glassware will not stand this temperature, a chemical disinfectant must be added to the second sink. Small glass-washing machines which can be fixed to the bar itself are often used in licensed premises. A sanitiser is added to the water and the cleaning action is performed by revolving brushes whilst the glass is held in place by hand. Machines with a separate rinsing chamber are preferable to single-chamber machines.

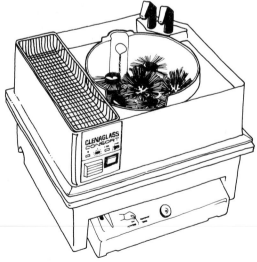

Glass-washing machine

The pan-wash

Pots, pans and other cooking vessels should be washed separately from crockery and cutlery. A tap proportioner can be fitted which will draw the correct amount of detergent from a container and mix it with the water. Scouring pads should be available. Stubborn grease can be removed by adding an alkali such as washing soda (sodium bicarbonate).

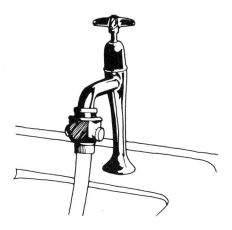

Tap proportioner

Storage containers

Particular care must be taken to wash thoroughly articles which are used for storage of food because if these are contaminated the bacteria will have time to multiply whilst food is being stored in them.

Working surfaces

Working surfaces should be cleaned as follows:

1. Wipe off crumbs and loose dirt.

2. Wash down with a detergent and water at a temperature of 50–60 °C (122–140 °F). Use disposable clothes or disinfect them daily.

3. Rinse thoroughly with a chemical disinfectant added to the water. This disinfectant solution must remain in contact with the surface for the time recommended in the instructions. Sanitisers (a detergent combined with a disinfectant) can be used for surfaces that are visibly clean, in which case stages 2 and 3 are combined.

Other equipment

A cleaning routine should be established for all large articles of equipment in use in the kitchen. As a general rule, all equipment which comes into direct contact with food should be cleaned after every use. Other surfaces and equipment should be cleaned as necessary. To ensure that cleaning is not overlooked it is a good idea to draw up a cleaning schedule which lists the items to be cleaned, the frequency and method of cleaning and the name of the person to whom the task is allotted.

HYGIENE SCHEDULE

All electrical appliances must be
switched off and disconnected

Frequency	Item	Method	Product	Allotted to
	Refrigerators and cold storage rooms	Brush or wipe all surfaces with disinfectant solution. Rinse with clean water and air-dry.		
	Floors	Apply disinfectant solution with clean string mop. Rinse. Air-dry.		
	Walls, doors and paintwork	Spray or sponge surfaces. Wipe clean with fresh, moist cloth. Air-dry.		
	Boilers and steamers	Scrub all surfaces with detergent. Rinse and air-dry. To descale: use recommended descaler. Rinse and air-dry.		
	Canopies	Spray or wipe surfaces with recommended detergent. Rinse and air-dry.		
	Tea/coffee urns	Scrub with recommended cleaning solution. Rinse thoroughly. Air-dry.		

Authorised by ....

Date ....

DISH-WASHING AT HOME

Few people have two sinks or a dish-washing machine at home so washing-up is not as conveniently done as in a large industrial kitchen. The temperatures used for washing with detergent and rinsing should be the same as in commercial premises. Rubber gloves will therefore be needed. After use, rubber gloves should be cleaned and dried.

It is important to remember that clean crockery and utensils can easily be recontaminated by a dirty tea towel. If tea towels are used for drying, it is essential that they are washed regularly. If the crockery and utensils are left to dry in the air they should be stacked away under cover as soon as they are dry and certainly before preparation and cooking of food begins again.

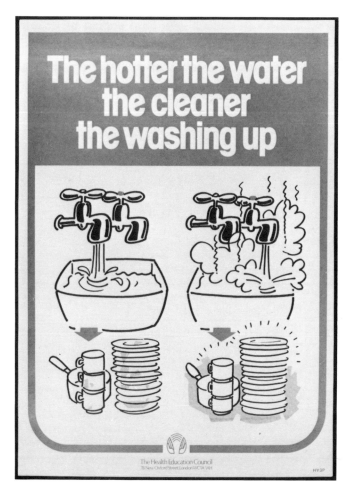

Health
Education
Council
poster

SUMMARY

1. Detergents remove dirt and grease but do not kill bacteria.

2. Disinfectants remove the majority of bacteria on surfaces and equipment.

3. Washing-up can be done by hand or machine. In both cases the articles to be cleaned are subjected to a detergent wash and are then rinsed in either hot water or water containing a chemical disinfectant.

4. Crockery and utensils should be covered and allowed to drain dry.

5. Glassware and pots and pans should be washed separately from the main wash.

6. Surfaces and equipment in contact with food should be cleaned after each use.

7. A cleaning schedule should be established for large equipment.

Chapter 16

Kitchen Design

It would be unrealistic for anyone to think that a kitchen can be made free from bacteria but there are several general principles concerning kitchen design and the layout of equipment which will help to reduce the risk of cross-contamination of foods. Apart from looking unpleasant, food crumbs, spillage from cooking, grease and dirt splashed on walls and on the floor, condensation on the ceiling and dust on window sills and floors will all be likely sources of pathogenic bacteria.

The main consideration in designing a kitchen is that the layout should allow easy cleaning and a continuous workflow from receiving raw foods through preparation and cooking to final presentation. Equipment should be movable or should be placed where it is possible to clean at the back, sides and underneath as well as at the front. If the equipment is not movable, it should, where possible, be built-in with one continuous surface between the equipment and the wall or floor so that dirt and grease cannot lodge in joints and corners.

A spacious kitchen is easier to keep clean and run hygienically than a small cramped kitchen. In a kitchen serving a restaurant, there must always be a division of preparation areas with the following points in mind:

1. Vegetable storage and preparation should be near to the delivery door. Potatoes and other vegetables have soil on them which carries *Cl. perfringens* spores and, if the vegetables are carried through the kitchen, dust from the vegetables may easily settle on cooked food.

2. Sections for raw meat preparation and cooked food preparation should be well separated to avoid cross-contamination because raw meat is frequently contaminated with *Salmonella* and *Cl. perfringens* bacteria.

3. The washing-up area should not be near the preparation areas so that dirty crockery and food waste will not come into contact with food to be eaten.

89

LIGHTING

In all kitchens it is essential that there is adequate lighting.

Natural light is less strain on the eyes than artificial light so windows should be large. Artificial light will of course be needed at times and should be bright enough to prevent accidents happening during food preparation and should be shadow-free so that all dirt is readily visible and the kitchen can be cleaned properly.

VENTILATION

Adequate ventilation in a kitchen is very important for two reasons:

1. To keep the temperature and humidity down. (The temperature and humidity of a hot steamy kitchen are ideal for bacterial growth.)
2. To remove cooking smells, steam, grease, etc.

    In a large industrial kitchen, hoods connected to extractor fans are usually fitted over the cookers. These must be cleaned regularly because grease and dirt reduce their efficiency.

    Windows which are opened for ventilation should be screened to prevent entry of insects and birds.

WORKING SURFACES

Working surfaces should be made from a hard-wearing easily cleaned material which will not absorb moisture, chip or crack, and will not be affected by food residues. Stainless steel is the usual choice. Wooden working surfaces should not be present as these rapidly become contaminated and are difficult to clean. Hardwood is still used for chopping boards but laminated plastic or compressed rubber boards are preferable. Different chopping boards must be used for preparing raw food and cooked food so that cross-contamination will not occur. Any surface which is chipped, cracked or badly scratched should be replaced as damaged surfaces will harbour food residues and hence bacteria.

WASTE DISPOSAL

Food waste is ideal for the growth of bacteria and unless it is carefully protected it will attract flies, rats, mice and other pests which may then transfer the bacteria back to fresh food in the kitchen.

Left-over food, residues from vegetable preparation such as potato peelings, and residues from other food preparation such as bones and gristle from meat should be removed from the working area immediately and put into pedal bins lined with plastic sacks or into disposable paper sacks with pedal-operated metal lids. There should be an adequate number of bins in the kitchen so that waste does not have to be carried across the kitchen. The bins must never be allowed to overflow and should be emptied regularly at the end of the day even if not full in order to remove a source of food for pests. It is essential to wash the hands after handling refuse and before handling food again.

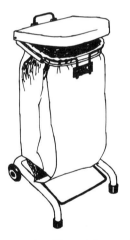

Paper sack with pedal-operated lid

A special area outside and not too near the kitchen window should be set aside for bins containing refuse and awaiting disposal. They should have tight fitting lids so that they cannot be knocked off by cats or dogs or blown off by the wind. An uncovered dustbin will attract flies and other insect pests, rats and mice. The bins should have rounded corners to facilitate cleaning and be placed on a metal stand approximately one foot above a drained and concreted area which should be washed down frequently.

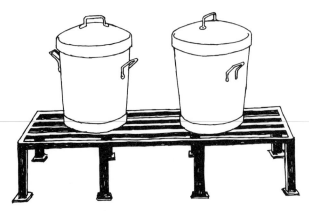

Dustbins — correct type and storage

Waste disposal units

These are a modern and convenient way of dealing with waste. They are made up of a system of high-speed cutters which shred the waste food which is then washed away into the drainage system.

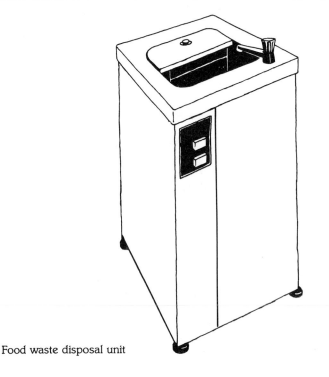

Food waste disposal unit

WASHING FACILITIES

Depending on the number of employees, an adequate number of hand-washing basins with hot and cold water, soap, a nailbrush and drying facilities must be present in convenient positions, e.g. at the entrance to the kitchen and next to the raw meat preparation areas. These must not be used for food preparation.

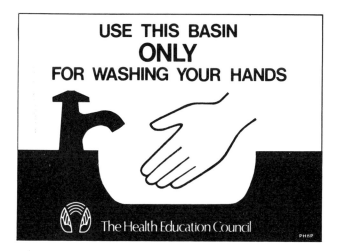

Stainless steel sinks should be located in each preparation area for washing food and must not be used for washing hands.

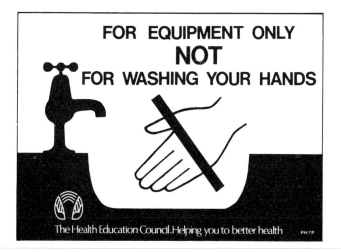

FLOORS

Kitchen floors should be made of a hard-wearing, anti-slip, easily cleaned material which will not absorb moisture and will not be affected by food residues such as grease, salt and fruit acids. Quarry tiles are popular but there are several other suitable materials available. There should be no breaks or cracks in the surface as these will allow dirt and bacteria to accumulate. The junction of the floor with the wall should be coved (rounded).

CEILINGS

Ceilings should have a smooth finish to facilitate cleaning. An absorbent plaster painted with a washable emulsion is often used. Gloss paint must not be used as it increases condensation. Polystyrene tiles are unsuitable because of the fire risk and because they are difficult to clean.

WALLS

Walls should have smooth surfaces which will be easy to clean and should be light-coloured to make dirt easily visible. Areas which frequently become soiled, e.g. around sinks and cooking apparatus, are best covered with ceramic tiles. Areas less susceptible to splashing can be painted with a gloss paint. Emulsion paint is too absorbent for this purpose.

SUMMARY

1. A well-planned, easily cleaned kitchen will save time and effort in food preparation and will reduce the risk of contamination of food.

2. The kitchen must be well lit and ventilated.

3. Floors, walls and working surfaces should be made from smooth, hard-wearing and non-absorbent materials.

4. An adequate number of hand-washing basins and food preparation sinks must be present.

5. Waste disposal units or disposable plastic or paper sacks which are removed from the kitchen regularly are the most hygienic methods of waste disposal.

Chapter 17

Kitchen Pests

Rats, mice, flies and cockroaches are the most common kitchen pests. Clean, well constructed and well maintained premises will not harbour any of these pests and it is therefore the duty of the food handler to make the premises where he works unattractive to pests by maintaining a high standard of hygiene.

RATS AND MICE

When rats and mice infest kitchens they are capable of causing considerable damage to food by gnawing through packets of food in storage and by eating almost any food which is easily accessible to them. The main problem is not the quantity of food pests eat but the amount they contaminate with harmful bacteria. Rats and mice frequently carry *Salmonella* in their intestines and so their droppings will contain live bacteria. They also carry bacteria on their fur and feet and can therefore transfer food poisoning bacteria from soil, waste food and refuse to uncovered food and surfaces used for food preparation just by running over them. Rats sometimes carry the bacterium that causes Weil's disease, an illness which gives rise to jaundice and can be fatal.

The need to wear down their continually growing incisor teeth means that rats and mice often gnaw woodwork, pipes and cables making costly repairs necessary. If they gnaw electric cables there is also a fire risk.

Rats and mice live and breed in warm dark corners where they will not be disturbed and where food is plentiful and easily accessible. To prevent infestation, food premises should be kept in good repair with no holes in the building and no defective pipes or drains, these being common means of entry for vermin. Pipe runs should be sealed at the entrance to buildings and wherever they pass from room to room.

Store rooms should be cleaned regularly. All stock must be kept off the ground and used in rotation to ensure that rats and mice are not being sheltered at the back of the store room.

Food should never be left uncovered in a kitchen and rubbish must not be allowed to accumulate inside or outside the building. All bins should have tight-fitting lids.

If any of the signs which indicate rodent infestation are noticed, such as gnawing marks, droppings or feet marks in dust or grain, measures to control it must be taken immediately because rodents breed prolifically. About 200 rats can develop from a pair and their young in a year, and given favourable conditions a pair of mice and their young can increase to 2000.

Many different poisons are effective in killing rats and mice but some of them are also poisonous to humans and domestic pets and are therefore not suitable for use in food premises. In the event of an infestation expert advice and treatment must be sought. The environmental health officer or a specialist organisation such as Rentokil should be contacted.

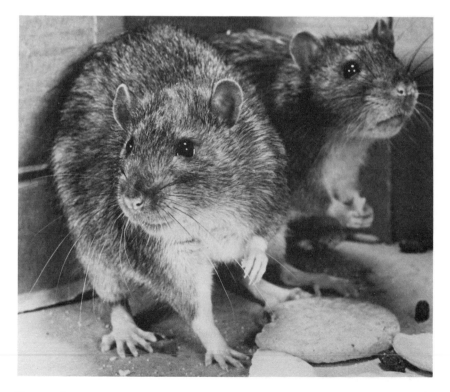

Brown rats

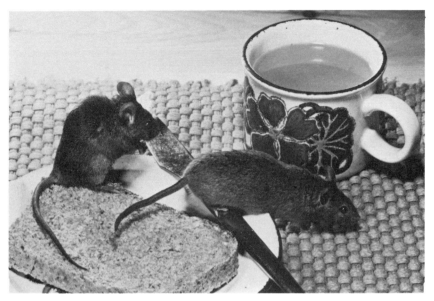

House mice

HOUSEFLIES AND BLUEBOTTLES

The number of flies in an urban environment has decreased significantly due to more efficient disposal of refuse and sewage. However, the housefly is still the commonest flying pest in buildings and its danger to health must not be underestimated. It feeds on refuse, from which it flies to human food where it deposits bacteria from its legs, wings, saliva and excrement.

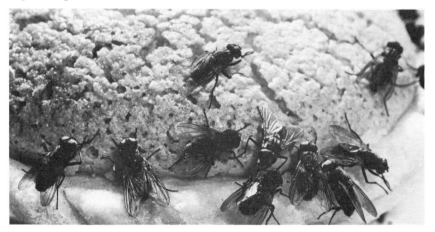

Houseflies

Flies breed very rapidly. They lay their eggs in warm, moist places such as on waste food and refuse. At summer temperatures it takes only ten days for the egg to develop into a maggot and then into an adult fly.

Bluebottles are characterised by their large size, their blue colour and the buzzing noise they make whilst flying. They are attracted to meat and fish products on which they lay their eggs.

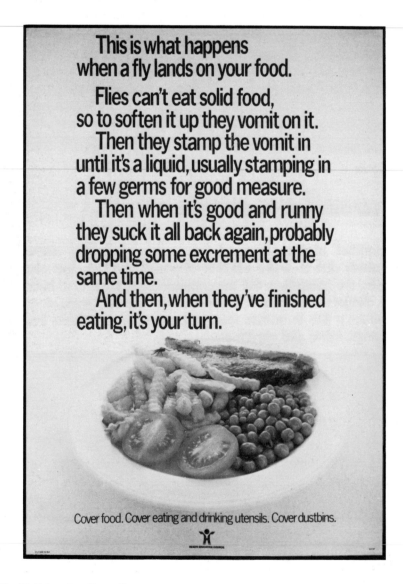

Health Education Council poster

The number of flies in a kitchen can be reduced by covering windows and ventilators with a gauze which is too fine to allow their entry. The use of mechanical waste disposal units also helps. If conventional bins are used, they should be kept firmly covered and regularly emptied and cleaned.

Insecticidal sprays must not be allowed to come into contact with food and therefore must not be used in rooms where food is prepared. Electrically operated fly killers are suitable for food preparation areas. They consist of an ultraviolet light which attracts flies to a metal grid with an electric current running through it. The flies are electrocuted when they touch the metal grid and fall into a collecting tray underneath.

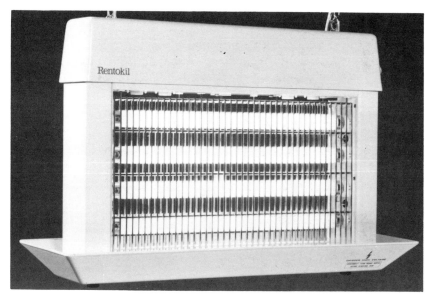

Electrically operated fly-killer

COCKROACHES

There are many different types of cockroach of varying sizes but only two are commonly found in the UK: the German cockroach and the oriental cockroach. The German cockroach is the smaller and is found in the kitchens of restaurants, hotels and industrial canteens. Typical hiding places are behind ovens and hot water pipes and around refrigerator motors. The larger oriental cockroach is usually found in the cooler and less humid parts of buildings such as basements, cellars and store rooms.

Their presence is not always detected at an early stage because they hide in crevices and cavities in the daytime and emerge to feed only at night. As they move around the kitchen in search of food they contaminate work surfaces, utensils, equipment and any uncovered food with pathogenic bacteria from their droppings and bodies.

An infestation by cockroaches can be recognised by their droppings and a characteristic and very unpleasant smell. It can be treated with insecticides but expert advice must be sought about their use in food premises. Several treatments will be necessary because the eggs of the cockroach are protected by a capsule and do not hatch out for several months.

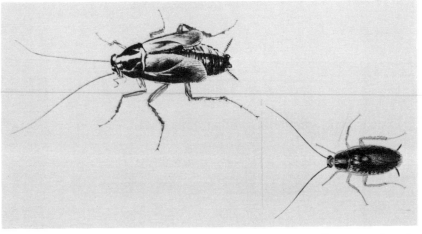

Oriental cockroach
(actual size 22 mm)

German cockroach
(actual size 12 mm)

SUMMARY

1. Rats, mice, flies and cockroaches are the most common kitchen pests.

2. Pests carry bacteria in their intestines, on their bodies and feet and can contaminate food or work surfaces with their droppings or by walking over them.

3. If an infestation of rats, mice or cockroaches is suspected, expert advice should be sought.

4. Electrically operated fly killers are the most satisfactory way of destroying flies in the kitchen.

Chapter 18

Other Diseases Spread by Food

There are many food-borne illnesses, several of which are far more serious than the food poisoning caused by *Salmonella, Staphylococcus aureus, Clostridium perfringens* and *Bacillus cereus*. Some are caused by bacteria. Others are caused by viruses, protozoa or parasitic worms (see Appendix 2).

BACTERIAL FOOD-BORNE DISEASES

These differ from bacterial food poisoning in that usually only a small number of bacteria need be present in the food in order to cause illness when it is eaten, whereas large numbers of bacteria must be present to cause the acute vomiting and diarrhoea known as food poisoning.

Bacterial food-borne diseases	Bacterial food poisoning
E.g. *Campylobacter* infection typhoid, paratyphoid, cholera, dysentery, brucellosis, tuberculosis	Caused by *Salmonella, Staphylococcus aureus, Cl. perfringens, B. cereus*
1. Relatively small numbers of the bacteria can cause illness.	1. Large numbers of the bacteria or toxins produced by them must be ingested before any ill effects are felt.
2. Time for multiplication in the food is not necessary.	2. Food must be left at a warm temperature for some time to allow the bacteria to multiply.
3. Infected drinking water frequently transmits these diseases.	3. Drinking water has never been known to be the cause of food poisoning.
4. The incubation period is fairly long: 1–25 days.	4. The incubation period is relatively short: 2–36 hours.

Food-borne diseases are frequently transmitted by contaminated drinking water, by food which has been washed in it, by shellfish or watercress gathered from it or by dehydrated food which has been rehydrated with it. After a natural disaster such as an earthquake or flooding, the drinking water sometimes becomes contaminated with sewage causing large outbreaks of these diseases.

Since the bacteria involved in food-borne diseases do not need time for multiplication in food, these diseases cannot be controlled by storage of food at the correct temperature. The food involved is merely a means of transport of the bacteria.

Campylobacter infection

Since 1977 there have been many reported outbreaks of diarrhoea which have been traced to certain species of the genus *Campylobacter*. These bacteria are now known to be the commonest cause of diarrhoea in the UK.

Incubation period	2–7 days
Symptoms	Flu-like symptoms for the first 24 hours, followed by abdominal pain, fever and diarrhoea which usually lasts from 1–5 days.
Cause of the disease	There is still much to be learnt about the cause of this disease. Many farm animals (cows, sheep and chickens) and domestic pets (cats, dogs) carry *Campylobacter* without showing any symptoms of illness. Some human infections are probably as a result of direct contact with these animals but most of the outbreaks have been traced to the consumption of unpasteurised milk and undercooked chicken. *Campylobacter* is not heat resistant and pasteurised milk and adequately cooked chicken have not caused any outbreaks.

Dysentery

There are two types of dysentery:

Bacillary dysentery is caused by several species of the genus *Shigella*. Outbreaks involving large numbers occur regularly in the UK.

Incubation period   1–7 days

Symptoms   Diarrhoea and fever. Sometimes vomiting.

Natural origin of the bacteria   *Shigella* is a parasite of man only and therefore if an outbreak occurs there must be a human carrier involved at some stage.

Causes of the disease

1. Personal contact. Bacillary dysentery can spread quickly in schools and institutions especially if personal hygiene standards are low (faecal-oral transmission).

2. Food handlers who are carriers of *Shigella* and have contaminated food by failing to wash their hands after a visit to the WC.

Amoebic dysentery   This disease is rare in Europe. It is caused by a protozoan (see p. 114).

Typhoid fever

Typhoid fever is caused by *Salmonella typhi*. It is a more severe form of illness than the food poisoning caused by the majority of species of the *Salmonella* genus. Typhoid fever is rare in the United Kingdom but occasionally people suffer on returning from a trip abroad. After the illness some people become convalescent carriers for the rest of their lives.

Incubation period   7–21 days

Symptoms   Prolonged fever with rose-coloured spots on the body. Severe diarrhoea usually commences in the second or third week of the fever. Typhoid fever is fatal in 2–10 per cent of all cases.

Natural origin of the bacteria   *Salmonella typhi* is a parasite of man only, unlike most other *Salmonellae* which are found in a wide variety of animals.

Causes of the disease

1. Food handlers who are carriers of *Salmonella typhi* and have con-taminated food by failing to wash their hands after a visit to the WC. People who are confirmed carriers of *Salmonella typhi* are not allowed to work in the food industry.

2. Drinking water that has been contaminated by sewage.

3. In a few instances, shellfish and watercress gathered from sewage-contaminated water have caused typhoid. Laws governing the gathering and cleansing of shellfish have more or less eliminated them as a cause of typhoid fever. Watercress should always be thoroughly washed.

Cholera

Cholera is a severe illness caused by a bacterium called *Vibrio cholerae*. It usually occurs as a result of eating food washed in sewage-contaminated water or by drinking the water itself. The symptoms are very severe diarrhoea and vomiting resulting in dehydration of the patient. The illness is often fatal and all visitors to countries where cholera is common should be vaccinated against it. Re-vaccination is required every six months.

Paratyphoid fever

Paratyphoid fever is caused by *Salmonella paratyphi*.

Incubation period   1–10 days

Symptoms   Fever, diarrhoea. Paratyphoid fever is similar to typhoid fever but the symptoms are generally less severe.

Natural origin of the bacteria   Human carriers.

Causes of the disease

1. Food handlers who are carriers of *Salmonella paratyphi*.

2. Drinking water that has been contaminated by sewage.

3. Food gathered from contaminated water.

SUMMARY

1. A food-borne disease caused by *Campylobacter* is the most common cause of diarrhoea in the UK.

2. Outbreaks of bacillary dysentery involving large numbers of people occur regularly in the UK.

3. Typhoid, paratyphoid and cholera are food-borne diseases which usually arise from the use of infected water.

Chapter 19

Food Hygiene Legislation

THE FOOD HYGIENE (GENERAL) REGULATIONS 1970

These regulations have been brought into force in order to protect public health and reduce the number of outbreaks of food poisoning. The number of the regulations is SI 1970 No. 1172 and copies can be bought either through a bookseller or direct from HMSO.

The regulations must be observed by anyone 'handling' food in a 'food business'.

The term 'food handler' includes anyone involved in the preparation or service of food and anyone involved in transport, storage, packing, wrapping and delivery of food.

The term 'food business' includes restaurants, cafés, canteens, boarding houses, food shops and food factories.

The Food Hygiene (General) Regulations 1970 can be divided into three main sections: PREMISES; PERSONAL HYGIENE; HYGIENIC PRACTICES.

PREMISES

1. *Buildings*   Buildings used as food premises should be clean and in good repair.

2. *Water supply*   Both hot and cold water must be available at each wash basin and at each sink used for washing food or equipment except where the sink is used *only* for a few special purposes such as washing fish, fruit or vegetables.

3. *Toilets*   Toilets must be clean, well lit and ventilated. A sufficient number of wash-basins must be provided and a 'Wash Your Hands' notice must be visible. The toilet must not open directly into a room where food is prepared or served.

4. *Washing facilities*   Wash basins must be kept clean and in good working order. An adequate supply of hot water, soap, nail brushes, clean towels or hot air driers must be provided.

5. *First aid kit*   Easily accessible bandages, dressings and antiseptics must be provided. Outer dressings should be waterproof.

6. *Clothing lockers for staff*   All staff must be provided with a locker where they can leave their outdoor clothing and footwear which is not used whilst working.

7. *Equipment*   Articles or equipment used for food preparation or storage must be kept clean and in good condition. Where possible they should be made of non-absorbent materials.

8. *Waste disposal*   Refuse must not be allowed to accumulate in a food room.

9. *Bedrooms*   A bedroom must not be used for food handling nor must it open directly into a food room. A food room must not be used as a sleeping place.

PERSONAL HYGIENE

Everyone handling food must observe certain hygiene precautions to prevent contamination of food.

1. *Cleanliness*   All parts of the person liable to come into contact with food (hands, forearms, face, hair and scalp) must be kept clean. Food handlers should avoid touching the nose and mouth and should wash their hands frequently.

2. *Clothing*   All personal clothing and overalls must be kept clean.

3. *Cuts and grazes*   All open cuts and grazes must be covered with a waterproof dressing.

4. *Smoking*   Smoking, spitting, chewing tobacco or using snuff is forbidden while handling food or while in a room where food is being handled.

5. *Personal health*   Food handlers must notify their employer at once if they are suffering from diarrhoea or vomiting, septic cuts, sores or boils. If the employer thinks they may be suffering from, or carriers of, typhoid fever, paratyphoid fever or any other *Salmonella* infection, dysentery or any Staphylococcal infection he must notify the local medical officer for environmental health who will decide whether or not the employee should stop handling food.

HYGIENIC PRACTICES

Prevention of contamination

1. *Cross-contamination* Raw and cooked food must be kept apart and different working surfaces and utensils must be used for their preparation.

2. *Storage* Food must not be placed out of doors within 40 cm (18 in) of the ground unless it is specially protected against contamination.

3. *Packaging* Food must not be packed in any container which might lead to contamination. Newspaper must not be used for wrapping food unless a clean inner wrapper is used as well.

4. *Animals* Live animals or live poultry must not be allowed to come into contact with food. Animal food must not be kept in a food room unless it is in a closed container.

Temperature control

Certain high-risk foods must not be stored at temperatures which will allow the rapid growth and multiplication of food-poisoning bacteria. Meat, game, poultry, fish, gravy and imitation cream and any foods prepared from them such as meat pies and fish patties, and also any foods made with egg, cream or milk such as cream cakes and trifle, must not be kept between the temperatures of 10 °C (50 °F) and 63 °C (145 °F) unless they are about to be served.

ENFORCEMENT OF REGULATIONS

The Food Hygiene Regulations are enforced by each local authority in its area and the environmental health department will give advice and guidance on them or on any aspect of food hygiene.

It is the legal responsibility of the manager of a food business to ensure that the required facilities are provided and used and that hygienic practices are observed at all times. Each individual food handler is responsible for complying with the regulations relating to personal hygiene.

If the medical officer for environmental health decides that a food handler is unfit to work for any of the reasons given under 5. *Personal health* (p. 106), the local authority will pay his wages for the period he is excluded from work. The food handler will, however, be prosecuted if he returns to work during that period.

Until February 1987 staff working in National Health Service premises had Crown immunity from prosecution if they contravened the Food Hygiene Regulations. This is no longer the case and NHS premises must now comply with all aspects of food hygiene legislation.

INVESTIGATION OF AN OUTBREAK OF FOOD POISONING

Any person who suspects that they are suffering from food poisoning should go to their doctor who is obliged to inform the medical officer for environmental health if he thinks his patient is suffering from food poisoning.

Outbreaks of food poisoning are investigated by a medical officer for environmental health together with an environmental health officer.

All patients are questioned about their symptoms, what food they have eaten in the last 48 hours and where it was eaten. Samples of their faeces are sent to a public health laboratory for bacteriological examination. If staphyloccal food poisoning is suspected, samples of vomit may be sent for analysis.

If most of the patients bought their food at a particular shop or restaurant, the environmental health officer will visit the premises and collect samples of any remaining suspect food. (Schools and hospitals keep sample meals in a refrigerator for several days after they have been served in case they are needed for examination.)

A faecal sample will be taken from anyone who is in contact with food at the premises, and if staphylococcal infection is suspected, nose, throat and skin swabs will be taken. Working surfaces and equipment may also be swabbed. All the samples are sent to the public health laboratory where they are checked to see whether they carry bacteria identical to those isolated from the patient.

If the cause of the outbreak is discovered, appropriate action will be taken to ensure that no further outbreaks occur. Food handlers who are found to be carriers will be excluded from work at least until they are free of symptoms. If inadequate temperature control or cross-contamination is responsible for the outbreak, advice will be given about storage and preparation of high-risk foods. Where unhygienic work surfaces or equipment are found to be the cause, advice will be given about appropriate cleaning programmes or replacement.

PROSECUTION AND CLOSURE OF PREMISES

The Food Act 1984 gives the environmental health officer (EHO) the power to enter and inspect all food premises and prosecute the owner or even close the premises if the Food Hygiene (General) Regulations 1970 are not being observed.

In most cases, rather than prosecution or closure and EHO will, after an inspection, send a notice specifying what needs to be done in order to comply with the regulations. A specified time limit is set for the necessary changes to be made.

For a particularly serious offence the local authority may decide to prosecute immediately. The maximum penalty for breach of the Food Hygiene Regulations is £2000.

If the EHO considers that the state of the premises means there is a significant risk of contamination of food the local authority will apply for a Closure Order. If there is also a serious risk to the health of customers they will apply for an Emergency Order. If the local authority wishes to apply for a Closure Order they must give the owner 14 days' written notice of their intention, specifying the changes required. They must give 3 days' written notice for an Emergency Order.

Where the application for a Closure Order or an Emergency Order is granted by the court, a copy of it is placed in a prominent place on the building.

In both cases, the premises may not be re-opened until the necessary improvements have been made. The EHO will inspect the premises again and if he finds them satisfactory a certificate allowing them to be re-opened will be issued within 14 days.

SUMMARY

1. The Food Hygiene (General) Regulations 1970 detail the legal requirements for food premises, the personal hygiene of staff and hygienic practices to be observed in food businesses.

2. Food poisoning outbreaks are investigated by an environmental health officer together with a medical officer for environmental health.

3. Food premises can be closed if the Food Hygiene Regulations are not observed.

Appendix 1

Further Causes of Food Poisoning

A few outbreaks of food poisoning are recorded each year which are attributed to causes other than those already described.

Vibrio parahaemolyticus

Vibrio parahaemolyticus is a comma-shaped bacterium. It is a common contaminant of fish and shellfish in tropical and subtropical waters. The few outbreaks of *V. parahaemolyticus* food poisoning which occur in the United Kingdom are usually traced to the consumption of imported seafood which has been contaminated after cooking (*V. parahaemolyticus* is sensitive to heat) and has been left unrefrigerated for some time.

The symptoms which usually occur between 12 and 18 hours after eating the contaminated food are abdominal pain and profuse diarrhoea often with vomiting and fever. The illness lasts from 2 to 5 days.

Although rare in Britain, *V. parahaemolyticus* is one of the most common causes of food poisoning in Japan.

Escherichia coli

Escherichia coli is a small rod-shaped bacterium. It is present in the intestinal tract of healthy people and is not normally pathogenic, but there are a few serotypes which are capable of causing diarrhoea in young children (usually under two years old). Adults are very rarely affected except when travelling abroad. 'Traveller's diarrhoea' is usually caused by a serotype of *E. coli* which is not found in the traveller's home country but may be widespread in the foreign country.

The symptoms which usually occur between 12 and 24 hours after eating the contaminated food are abdominal pain, fever, diarrhoea and sometimes vomiting. The illness lasts from 1–5 days.

E. coli is used as an indicator organism in food analysis. The presence of *E. coli* in food suggests that the food has at some stage been contaminated from a faecal source and therefore implies that there is a potential risk of the presence of more harmful intestinal organisms such as *Salmonella*.

Yersinia enterocolytica

Yersinia enterocolytica is a rod-shaped bacterium which can grow slowly at refrigeration temperatures. Some strains appear to cause food poisoning in Britain. The main symptom, which occurs 24–36 hours after consumption of the infected food, is diarrhoea, sometimes accompanied by abdominal pains, fever and vomiting.

Scombrotoxic fish poisoning

Scombrotoxic fish poisoning was first reported in the United Kingdom in 1976 and since then there have been several incidents as a result of the consumption of mackerel, tuna, sardines or pilchards.

The illness is caused by toxins which accumulate in the flesh of the fish during unrefrigerated storage. The fish do not always appear spoilt but analysis of them reveals a higher level of histamine than would be found in fresh fish. The presence of high levels of histamine (derived from the amino acid histidine) is not thought to be the cause of symptoms, only an indicator that the fish may be poisonous.

The toxin is not easily destroyed by heat and freshly opened canned fish has caused some of the outbreaks.

Symptoms occur between 15 minutes and 3 hours after eating the fish and include a burning sensation in the mouth, flushing, urticaria, headache, nausea, vomiting and diarrhoea. They last for up to 8 hours.

Paralytic shellfish poisoning

Paralytic shellfish poisoning occurs only rarely in the United Kingdom but it is a serious and sometimes fatal type of food poisoning. It can occur following the consumption of mussels and other bivalves which have been feeding on a certain type of plankton which produces a neurotoxin.

Symptoms occur between ½ and 3 hours after eating the fish and include a tingling of the tongue and mouth which spreads to the neck, fingers and toes and occasionally progresses to paralysis. A large outbreak occurred in 1968 involving mussels, and since then annual monitoring of the toxin levels in mussels has taken place.

Appendix 2

Further Food-borne Diseases

BACTERIAL

Listeriosis

Outbreaks of listeriosis are becoming more common. *Listeria monocytogenes* is widely distributed in the environment and is found in soil, water and sewage. Foods which are known to have caused Listeriosis are cole-slaw, fresh salad, milk, soft cheese and chicken.

Listeriosis can cause meningitis, septicaemia and, in pregnant women, miscarriage or stillbirth. Only a small proportion of people eating contaminated food shows symptoms. The incubation period can be as long as 4 weeks.

Listeria monocytogenes can grow at refrigeration temperatures and is therefore a potential problem in cook-chill foods. It is likely that the guidelines relating to this method of food preparation will be reviewed in the near future.

Brucellosis and tuberculosis

These two diseases are usually spread by contaminated milk. Since the introduction of pasteurisation of milk, they have become rare. Pasteurisation is a heating process which ensures that all pathogenic bacteria are destroyed although some spoilage bacteria and other non-pathogenic bacteria may remain alive.

Brucellosis (Undulant fever) is caused by a bacterium called *Brucella abortus*.

Incubation period	5–21 days
Symptoms	Variable but usually pain in muscles and joints and a fever. The disease is rarely fatal but can give rise to prolonged ill health.

Tuberculosis is caused by a species of the genus *Mycobacterium.*

Incubation period   4–6 weeks

Symptoms   The bovine type affects the bones, lymph nodes and intestines and is usually caused by drinking unpasteurised milk from infected cattle. The other type affects the lungs and is airborne. Both types of tuberculosis, though rare now, were common diseases in the early part of this century.

Control of brucellosis and tuberculosis.

1.   Cattle herds are now checked regularly to ensure that they are free from these diseases. Infected animals are slaughtered.

2.   Pasteurisation of milk.

VIRAL

Hepatitis

The strict meaning of hepatitis is inflamed liver. There are three types of viral hepatitis: hepatitis A; hepatitis B and non A/non B hepatitis. Of these, only hepatitis A is transmitted by food.

Hepatitis A: This form of hepatitis accounts for 70 per cent of all cases. The incubation period is long (about 28 days) and the symptoms are fever, nausea, abdominal pain and, later, jaundice. The 'duration' of the illness can be anything from a week to several months and the severity of the symptoms varies considerably. Many children suffer a mild gastro-intestinal disturbance but do not become jaundiced. However, this mild illness will give them life-long immunity.

The virus is spread by the faecal-oral route and so food can be contaminated by a food handler with poor hygiene standards who is a carrier of the virus. The majority of food-borne outbreaks have been associated with shellfish collected from sewage-contaminated waters. Milk also has been implicated.

Hepatitis B: The symptoms are similar to hepatitis A but more severe. Transmission is by contact with infected blood or other body fluids.

Non A/Non B hepatitis: This is a collective term for any cases of viral hepatitis except hepatitis A and hepatitis B. The major source of these infections is from blood transfusions.

PROTOZOAL

Protozoa are single-celled micro-organisms. They live in an aqueous (watery) environment, e.g. soil saturated with water, ponds, ditches, rivers and the sea. The majority are harmless but a few are pathogenic to man.

Giardiasis

Giardiasis is caused by the protozoan *Giardia lamblia.* The illness occurs world-wide but is more common in areas of poor sanitation, the main source of infection being human carriers.

The incubation period is 1–4 weeks and the predominant symptom is profuse watery diarrhoea often accompanied by abdominal pain and nausea. The severity of the symptoms varies and children, although more frequently infected, tend to suffer less than adults.

Direct person to person transmission via the faecal-oral route is the most common means of spread. Water or food may also be contaminated.

Amoebic dysentery

Amoebic dysentery is caused by the protozoan *Entamoeba hystolytica.* The disease is spread by the faecal-oral route or from contaminated water or food. The incubation period is usually 3–4 weeks and the main symptoms are abdominal pain and diarrhoea.

Although rare in Europe it is endemic in some tropical countries particularly where sanitation and hygiene are primitive and faecal contamination of the environment is common.

Cryptosporidium

The protozoan *Cryptosporidium* is known to cause many cases of gastro-enteritis. The main symptoms are profuse watery diarrhoea, abdominal pain and fever which last for about 10 days. It is usually spread by the faecal-oral route but it is thought that some cases may have occurred as a result of drinking contaminated milk since *Cryptosporidium* can survive the process of pasteurisation.

PARASITIC WORMS

Tapeworms

These are flat worms consisting of a head and a chain of flat oblong segments arising from the headpiece. There are two types of tapeworm: one is found in cattle and the other in pigs. In both instances cysts settle in the muscle of the infected animal giving the meat a spotted appearance which can usually be detected when the meat is inspected. If infected meat is eaten the cysts develop in the human intestine into tapeworms which can grow to several feet in length.

The symptoms are abdominal pain, increased appetite and loss of weight because the tapeworm takes in digested food before the infected person has time to absorb it. Worm infections in the UK are very rare since meat is inspected before distribution.

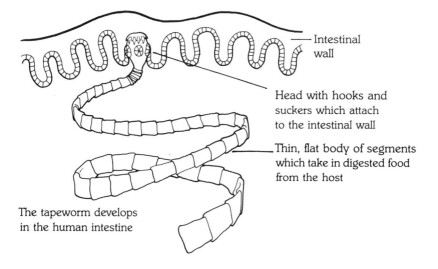

Intestinal wall

Head with hooks and suckers which attach to the intestinal wall

Thin, flat body of segments which take in digested food from the host

The tapeworm develops in the human intestine

Trichinosis

Trichinosis is caused by the worm *Trichinella spiralis*. The disease is transmitted by meat, usually pork. Cysts settle in the muscle of infected animals. If the meat is inadequately cooked the cysts will survive, and when the meat is eaten they will develop in the human body into small worms.

The symptoms of trichinosis are abdominal pain, muscular pain, swelling of the eyelids and pain around the eyes.

Trichinosis is very rare in the UK due to routine meat inspection but it is a wise precaution to cook pork thoroughly.

Examination Questions

Chapter 1
1. Are all bacteria harmful? Describe the effects which different types of bacteria have on food.

Chapter 2
1. What are the four requirements for bacterial growth? Write a short paragraph about each one.
2. Write notes on:
   (a) Spores.
   (b) Foods which are susceptible to bacterial growth.
   (c) Anaerobes.
3. Describe the conditions which make bacteria dormant.

Chapter 3
1. Write notes on:
   (a) Incubation periods for bacterial food poisoning.
   (b) Chemical food poisoning.
   (c) Vegetable food poisoning.
   (d) Viral food poisoning.

Chapter 4
1. Explain what is meant by cross-contamination. If you owned a butcher's shop what advice would you give to your staff to prevent this occurring?
2. In what ways are pathogenic bacteria spread to food?
3. What are (a) healthy carriers and (b) convalescent carriers? What could be the result of a 'carrier' working in a food preparation area?

Chapter 5
1. What precautions would you take when preparing food to prevent *Salmonella* food poisoning arising?
2. Which bacterium causes the majority of food poisoning outbreaks? How is it usually spread into foods?

Chapter 6
1. If you were in charge of preparing sandwiches for a self-service counter, what precautions would you take to ensure that food poisoning due to *Staphylococcus aureus* did not occur?
2. Explain why a food can cause bacterial food poisoning even if there are no live bacteria in it?

Chapter 7
1. Why is the bacterium *Clostridium perfringens* particularly difficult to destroy? What precautions can you take to prevent this type of food poisoning occurring?
2. How is *Clostridium perfringens* usually brought into the kitchen? What would be a typical chain of events leading to this type of food poisoning?

Chapter 8
1. Why is food poisoning due to *Clostridium botulinum* the most dangerous form of food poisoning and under what conditions can it occur?

Chapter 9
1. Why is it particularly important that meat products and rice should not be reheated more than once?

Chapter 10
1. Why is it particularly important to maintain a high standard of personal hygiene when preparing food?
2. Write what you know about the following:
   (a) The hand-washing facilities which must, by law, be provided for food handlers.
   (b) The advantages and disadvantages of the various methods of hand-drying.
   (c) The occasions when hands must be washed.

Chapter 11
1. Give reasons for the following statements:
   (a) 'Thaw frozen meat completely before cooking.'
   (b) 'Keep food either very hot or very cold.'
2. Describe the common faults in food preparation which frequently contribute to outbreaks of food poisoning.

Chapter 12
1. Which foods should always be stored in a refrigerator and why? How would you position the foods you have mentioned in the refrigerator?
2. Why are refrigerators important in the prevention of food poisoning? How can you ensure that the temperature of the refrigerator is maintained?

3. Why can food be kept for a longer period of time in a freezer than in a refrigerator? What would you do if your freezer broke down?
4. Write a short description of the cook-chill and cook-freeze methods of food preparation.

Chapter 13
1. What types of food do not normally support the growth of food poisoning bacteria? In each case explain briefly why this is so.
2. Made-up meat dishes are frequently a cause of food poisoning. Give reasons for this.
3. Make a list of milk and dairy products which are often used in the kitchen and give reasons why some of them may cause food poisoning and others normally do not.

Chapter 14
1. What are the principal reasons for the increase in the number of outbreaks of food poisoning in the UK?
2. Why are there more outbreaks of food poisoning during the summer months than during the winter months?

Chapter 15
1. In a restaurant serving 100 meals each evening, describe how you would organise the washing-up if you did not have a dish-washing machine.
2. Describe the different functions of detergents and disinfectants and their importance in preventing food poisoning.

Chapter 16
1. If you were asked to plan a new kitchen what points regarding the design and layout would you consider important?
2. Why is efficient waste disposal important in the prevention of food poisoning?

Chapter 17
1. What indications might there be of an infestation by rats or mice? What action would you take?
2. What are the most common kitchen pests? How can they cause food poisoning?
3. What steps can you take to reduce the risk of an infestation of pests in your food premises?

Chapter 18
1. Explain what is meant by 'bacterial food-borne diseases.' How do these differ from food poisoning?

Chapter 19
1. Give a brief summary of The Food Hygiene (General) Regulations 1970 under the following headings:
   (a) Premises.
   (b) Personal hygiene.
   (c) Hygienic practices.
2. An outbreak of food poisoning has occurred among school children. How would this outbreak be investigated?
3. What powers does the Food Act 1984 give to an environmental health officer concerning food premises?

General
1. 'Food poisoning will occur only if food is prepared in dirty premises.' Discuss this statement.
2. What would you include in a lecture on food hygiene to a group of hospital caterers?
3. Which of the following foods particularly favour the growth of food poisoning bacteria and which rarely do? Explain why.
   (a) A 'rare' steak.
   (b) Stuffed, rolled breast of lamb.
   (c) Fried rice.
   (d) A cheddar cheese sandwich.
4. What hand-washing facilities must, by law, be provided in food premises and why?
5. What are the reasons for not allowing pets into food premises?
6. Write notes on three of the following:
   (a) Methods of waste disposal.
   (b) Materials suitable for use as working surfaces.
   (c) Lighting and ventilation in kitchens.
   (d) Keeping the kitchen free of flies.
7. 'Provided that food is hot, it is safe to eat.' Discuss this statement.
8. Which raw foods frequently carry food poisoning bacteria? How can cross–contamination be prevented?
9. Write briefly about three bacteria which commonly cause food poisoning in Britain.

10. Write notes on four of the following:
    (a) *Vibrio cholerae.*
    (b) *Clostridium botulinum.*
    (c) *Salmonella typhi.*
    (d) *Campylobacter.*
    (e) *Shigella.*
11. You have decided to go on a day trip in the car with some friends. You will be leaving early in the morning, stopping for lunch at a restaurant and packing a picnic tea. When deciding what to take, what points would you bear in mind to prevent food poisoning occurring?
12. Describe the food hygiene precautions you would take if organising a wedding reception for one hundred people to be held under canvas in June.

Royal Society of Health examination questions
Taken from the RSH certificate examination in the hygiene of food retailing and catering.

1. List three ways in which food may become contaminated in a kitchen.
2. List the three main conditions necessary for encouraging the growth of bacteria in foods.
3. Does the appearance of food normally indicate the presence of food poisoning organisms?
4. What food poisoning organism is frequently associated with pre-cooked meat meals?
5. (a) Above what temperature should foods that are to be kept hot be stored?
   (b) Below what temperature should foods that are to be kept cold be stored?
6. What should a food handler do in the following circumstances:
   (a) If a finger is cut.
   (b) If suffering from sickness and diarrhoea?
7. Why should poultry be defrosted before cooking?
8. What do you understand by the term 'incubation period' with respect to food poisoning?
9. State precisely the meaning of cross-contamination.
10. If a member of the public became ill with acute vomiting shortly after consuming a Chinese meal containing rice, which food poisoning organism would you suspect?
11. List the high-risk protein foods.

12. Give two reasons why a kitchen must be well ventilated.
13. What action could an environmental health officer take if he/she found premises which were so dirty as to be a risk to public health?
14. What would lead you to suspect that your premises were infested with rats?
15. Briefly describe the 'two-sink system' of dish-washing.
16. What is a tap proportioner?
17. What is the title of the legislation which regulates hygiene in all food premises?
18. What is a pathogen?
19. What is a carrier?
20. What comments can you make on the practice of placing the 'sweets' trolley in a restaurant dining room throughout the evening?
21. State three important rules which should always be remembered when using a refrigerator.
22. Which harmful bacteria are most likely to be transferred to food by a food handler who bites his/her finger nails?
23. Why is it considered unwise to stuff a chicken before it is cooked?
24. Why are rolled joints of meat less safe than solid joints of meat?
25. What are the three most important precautions to undertake when preparing poultry in a kitchen?
26. Name two diseases other than food poisoning that may be transmitted by food.
27. What is the recognised maximum keeping time for 'cook-chill' foods?
28. Statistics show that food poisoning is on the increase. Give two causes for this increase.
29. Frozen food manufacturers use star markings on packages to provide the consumer and others with storage life information. Give the storage life and equivalent temperature for the following:
    (a) one star. *1 week*
    (b) two stars. *1 month*
    (c) three stars. *3 months.*
30. If frozen food defrosts, is it good practice to refreeze it?

GCE Advanced level domestic science and home economics examination questions

1. What is food poisoning and how is it caused? When does food poisoning constitute a real danger to life?
    Consider the implications of a chef with a heavy cold preparing dishes for the sweet trolley.
    (The Associated Examining Board, June 1985)

2. Describe the ways in which bacterial food poisoning may be caused. Comment on the fact that food handlers need to use all the knowledge they can acquire to help reduce the incidence of food poisoning.
    (The Associated Examining Board, June 1984)

3. Compare the properties of the materials used to make the following and say how those properties affect the use and care of the equipment in each case.
    (a) An enamelled sink and a stainless-steel sink.
    (b) A wooden chopping board and a laminated plastic chopping board.
    (c) Vinyl floor tiles and quarry tiles in an institutional kitchen.
    What general principles of design should be incorporated in equipment in order to make its use and cleaning as easy and as effective as possible?
    Evaluate the contribution to efficient and safe working that good lighting and ventilation systems can make in a canteen kitchen.
    (The Associated Examining Board, June 1983)

4. Begin each sentence with the name of the appropriate micro-organism:
    (a) _Staphaurea_ is found in the nasal cavity of many individuals and can cause food poisoning.
    (b) _C. Colulus_ survives inadequate canning or bottling and may cause death.
    (c) _Salmonella_ exists in poultry and survives inadequate cooking to cause food poisoning.
    (University of London, June 1984)

5. Name three of the chief micro-organisms responsible for outbreaks of food poisoning and suggest two potential sources of each.
    (University of London, June 1983)

Index